How to END a LIFE

How to END a LIFE

A DEATH PANEL STORY

ANTONIO ARATA

To Nancy –
My strength,
my encouragement,
and my love.

LIFE (OR AS WE ONCE KNEW IT)

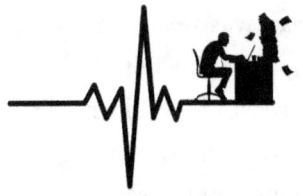

INTRODUCTION

Staring at the medical chart on the computer screen, Evan Coleman couldn't help but think about his first kill. Oh, it wasn't like that. There was no weapon, no malice, nor even a motive. But a kill, nonetheless.

He'd never forget her. Constance Roth. Seventy-three years old. Half-blind, mostly deaf, yet still living alone on the outskirts of town. No family, no contributions to society. So many comorbidities that it was comical. Heart disease, diabetes, seventy-four kilograms over the allowed weight set by D-MACS for her height, rheumatoid arthritis, enlarged liver, history of stroke and myocardial infarctions. And bunions. Why the hell did they throw in bunions? Evan laughed every time he thought about it. Maybe it was meant to add some levity to the job. Who knew?

Evan had never met her. The panel wasn't allowed to. If you never met the person, heard their story, or looked into their eyes, then the decision was less stressful. Such was the thought, anyway.

It was an easy kill. The panel had unanimously agreed

upon her fate. With seven voting members and two alternates, a complete consensus was rare. Yet Ms. Roth never had a chance.

The chart Evan was reviewing now, however, was less cut and dry. Many times, he felt like he had been duped into believing every case would be like his first. Poor Ms. Roth.

"Hurry up, putz. I'm not staying one extra minute this time because of your dumb ass."

Evan could always count on Murray to keep him on task. Loud. Obnoxious. Way too much aftershave and not enough deodorant. Perpetually single yet naively optimistic. And now a clock-watcher to boot. Great qualities in a coworker.

"I'll have my reviews done and tabbed by five o'clock, don't worry, Murr."

Murray belched a combination of processed pork and diet coke in Evan's direction. "You better. I'm meeting Rita for drinks at Marketside and I will not be late for our second date. That's right. I said second. You got a problem with that?"

Evan raised his eyebrows.

"Nope. Sounds great. Let me crank out my charts so you won't be late."

Evan returned his attention to the computer screen. Even though D-MACS had written actuary code years ago to calculate an aggregate score, every member of the panel still reviewed each chart to make the final determination. Mr. Hank Isley had scored a sixty-six, as any moron could see. But what D-MACS's code writers couldn't capture were the subtle intricacies of what a panelist needed to make a final judgment. And Evan was the best of the best at making final judgments. Much to the dismay of a Mr. Hank Isley, number 5034928.

"Sorry, Hank," Evan whispered. "You should have taken better care of yourself when you had a chance."

Evan didn't hesitate as he selected the "REJECT" button. Why couldn't making the judgment of Ms. Roth been as easy? Her review was obvious to all, but his nervousness at making the wrong decision paralyzed him with fear. He recalled holding the cursor over the "REJECT" button for Ms. Roth for a full ten minutes then.

Oh, what a difference a decade made.

TIME IN A BOTTLE

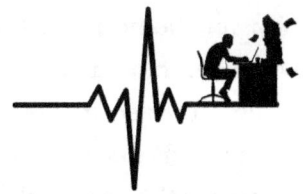

CHAPTER ONE

Leo McGregor loved life. Though not too bright, he had enough sense when the situation called for it. Like when his neighbors, the Flemings, were away on their annual Grand Canyon vacation and Leo was asked to keep an eye on their place. Anybody could call 9-1-1 and wait for the fire department to show up when the Fleming's cat chewed its way through the sofa lamp, creating a spark which set the couch on fire. Not Leo. Thanks to his quick thinking and creative use of a garden hose (and the Fleming's above-ground pool), by the time the volunteer fire department made it, the only damage found was to an algae-soaked couch left smoldering in the homestead.

Or the time when Luanne, Leo's wife of thirty-three years, turned blue while choking on the Thanksgiving turkey. While the rest of the McGregor clan remained paralyzed in terror, Leo didn't even put down his drumstick to administer the Heimlich maneuver. Once the expectorated turkey was safely dislodged into Luanne's lap, he simply grabbed the gravy boat and returned to his seat. Hey, Leo loved life,

5

and he made the most of each day.

However, the day the aneurysm ruptured, turning Luanne's ascending aorta into a burst balloon, Leo finally met his match. They were home alone, the McGregor children having grown up and moved out years ago, when the pain hit Luanne. She screamed before collapsing on the floor of the patio where moments before Leo had been beating her in a heated game of Rummy. With his wife's propensity for being overly dramatic, Leo's first thought was that she was upset about losing at cards (again) and was trying to make him feel bad.

It would not have been the first time. When Leo had finally had enough of his mother-in-law's overextended visits every summer, Luanne faked Lupus with a twist of Lyme disease, necessitating the need for her mother to stay for a couple more weeks to convalesce her back to health.

Leo stared at Luanne for a full minute before realizing this was not one of her Academy Award winning performances but, instead, a true medical emergency. The EMTs were able to get a pulse back before loading her into the ambulance and whisking her away.

Then it got weird for Leo.

Having spent years watching medical shows and an occasional "Healthy Minute" interruption during a sports game (well, he could hear the infomercial through the door to the bathroom sometimes), Leo thought he knew what to expect at Regional General Hospital, where Luanne was rushed by the EMTs. So sure of what would happen, Leo didn't think it'd be too out of line to stop off at the local Fill 'Er Up on the way to the hospital to top off the truck's tank. And, while there, he might as well grab a roller dog and a Dew for the road. Who knew how long it'd be before he'd get something else to eat if he had to stay at the hospital with Luanne.

Leo did some quick figuring. "Let's see, on most medical shows, the doctor sees the patient in the emergency room, runs some tests, has a quick fling in the supply closet with a cute intern, and then starts the discharge paperwork before the hour is up."

Thinking about how fast this always happened, he scarfed down the snack and sped off, convinced that the sexually sated physician would be writing the last prescription at the exact moment Leo would walk into the hospital.

"Hmmmm ..." Leo said to himself. On a couple of them medical dramas, the cute female intern sometimes hit on the doting husband almost immediately. After pulling into Regional General's parking lot, Leo splashed on some Old Spice he kept in the glove box ... just in case. Turned out, much to Leo's surprise (which quickly morphed to confusion) upon walking into the emergency department, the antiquated cologne was not necessary. Luanne was not sitting up on the side of a gurney, getting final discharge instructions from a perfectly coiffed, two-day stubbled, part-time model/full-time doctor. Luanne was nowhere in sight. In fact, no other patients were in sight either. Just an empty emergency department with one triage station, one triage nurse, and one transporter leaning casually against the one lone stretcher.

Then it got weirder for Leo.

"Welcome to Regional General Hospital," the triage nurse said to Leo when he walked up to the desk. She languidly looked up from her magazine. "How can I help you?"

Confused, Leo stammered out, "Ummm, well, my wife collapsed at home a little while ago, and the EMTs said they were bringing her here, ..." Leo trailed off, peering beyond the triage nurse, trying to see something, anything, of what was going on in this place.

The triage nurse heaved a bored sigh. "I can try to help you. What's your wife's name?"

As soon as Leo said "Luanne McGregor," the nurse darted her eyes to the transporter, who nodded in recognition.

"Of course, Mrs. McGregor," she said, typing into the laptop on her desk. "She came in twenty-five minutes ago and was taken to the back to be evaluated by the D-MACS team. If you'll have a seat, I'll let the lead evaluator know you're here." At this, the nurse entered more information into the computer, closed the laptop, and smiled at Leo. "Please, have a seat over there." She waved to a small waiting room with six chairs in it.

Leo sat down, rubbing his temples. None of the shows he watched (and none of the partial health updates he almost heard from the bathroom) had indicated hospitals could become empty rooms, devoid of hustle, absent of bustle, and, most strikingly, bereft of patients.

What the hell was a lead evaluator, anyway? Why was he not meeting with a doctor? His eyes landed on posters taped to the wall.

"YOUR HEALTH IS OUR GOAL!" the colorful poster proclaimed over a picture of a typical doctor in a lab coat and stethoscope, kicking a soccer ball full force into a net.

"D-MACS—KEEPING YOU IN THE HEALTH LANE," another poster announced, with an animated, cartoonish D-MACS monolith driving a convertible down a freeway toward a sunset.

"Well," thought Leo as he considered both posters for several minutes, "maybe Luanne is in the right place after all." The soccer-ball-kicking, goal-winning doctor did have the appearance of a lead in the medical dramas. "I'm sure the cute intern will show up any minute," Leo hoped, checking the aroma of his go-to aftershave.

Instead, a man in his thirties, with a short sleeve shirt, stiff tie, and nervous smile came into the waiting area. "Mr. McGregor. I'm Carl Duncan, assistant lead evaluator for D-MACS here at Regional General. Can you come with me please?"

Gnawing on his lip, Leo stood up and followed the man out of the small waiting room and into another, smaller room with only a metal table and two chairs, one of which was occupied by another thirty-something-year-old man. He wore short sleeves as well but with a noticeably stiffer tie and a less-nervous smile. Averting his gaze from the computer monitor in front of him, the man stood and shook Leo's hand. "Bill Wilson," he said, offering him a seat at the table.

Carl leaned toward Leo. "Would you care for anything? Water? Coffee?"

Annoyed, Leo replied, "No, but I'd take a heaping cup of 'what-the-hell-is-going-on?'"

Carl feebly smiled back at Leo.

Bill steepled his fingers. "Precisely what I'm here to do, Mr. McGregor. I know you must be confused, and I am here to answer all your questions. Please. Have a seat."

"I'll give the two of you some privacy," Carl announced,

casting a knowing glance towards Bill. "I'm just outside the door if you should need anything."

As Carl left the room, Leo sat down in the chair next to the lead evaluator's desk. The computer monitor was turned slightly, offering Leo a glimpse at the screen. Gasping, he was surprised to see an image of what appeared to be his wife— looking quite dead—and lying on hospital gurney. Despite his eyes watering, Leo couldn't turn away from the image.

Bill quickly minimized the screen, pulling up a page with a D-MACS logo, something like a questionnaire form by appearances. "Mr. McGregor, in order for us to help your wife, we need some information."

Sniffling, Leo said, "You mean ... I mean ... she ain't dead? That picture I just saw on your computer ..."

Without hesitation, Bill jumped in. "Oh no, no ... your wife is currently under the expert care of the Regional General medical team. We need information from you in order to best determine the plan of treatment for her. As you can guess, D-MACS must have up-to-date health information prior to treatment. Thus, time is of the essence. Are you ready?"

Leo nodded, prompting the tedious process of answering no fewer than ninety-seven questions about Luanne's hobbies, preferences, habits, ideologies, work history, favorite movies and music, thoughts, dreams, and greatest accomplishments. Not until questions eighty-four through ninety-seven, was he asked about her actual health history. Leo did his best to answer each one but, after thirty-three years of marriage, how much did anyone really know about their wife?

Bill, who had been entering Leo's answers into the computer, tapped a key with flair and leaned back.

"Thank you, Mr. McGregor. You did wonderfully. Your answers will help the team to decide the next steps to best assist your wife. Well done ... well done." Bill had an unreadable poker face though his voice sounded reassuring, optimistic even. "We are going to do all we can."

Leo scratched his jaw. "I'm still not sure what's going on here. Neither of us has seen a doctor in about fifteen years, and you haven't even told me what's wrong with Luanne or what is going to happen now. Where is the doctor? Where is Luanne?"

"Your wife had a dissection, or tear, of her aorta— the large blood vessel that takes oxygen-rich blood to smaller blood vessels, which then deliver the blood to your organs. The tear was quite substantial, and the medical team is doing everything they can."

Leo pressed for more answers. "Is she going to surgery? Can it be repaired?"

"The team is evaluating this now. They needed the health history first to know how to best help her next."

"You needed to know she hasn't worked in thirteen years because of a back injury and that she likes Chinese food every Friday night to determine whether or not surgery would help her?" Leo asked, his anger rising.

"Mr. McGregor. I know this must seem confusing. Yes, the medical team needs to know this information. Every clue to your wife's health can be elicited by the questions I asked you. For example, your wife's chronic back pain could have been her body telling her that she had signs of an aneurysm for quite a while. And weekly consumption of MSG is unsafe for those with high blood pressure, which your wife has a history of. So, as you can see, these questions do have a purpose."

Leo immediately shrank back in his chair, embarrassed to have questioned the obvious medical expertise and care of this evaluator. *Of course they are here to help her. That's what they do.*

"I'm sorry I questioned you, Mr. Wilson. Thank you. Thank you for explaining, and thank you for doing everything for my Luanne."

"Of course, Mr. McGregor. Now if you'll have a seat back in the first waiting room, I need to confer with my colleagues about next steps in your wife's care."

Leo stood and shook Bill's hand before walking back to the small waiting room.

Carl immediately entered the office and sat down across from Bill. "Wow. That's all I can say. Wow."

"You heard all that?" Bill said, eyebrows quirked.

"Did I? Where did you come up with the MSG line? It was classic!"

"I thought I heard it somewhere. Anyway, he seemed to buy it." Bill smugly smiled. He had once again navigated his way out of a landmine situation (irate husband) back to the realm of trust.

"You're the best, Bill. Every day I learn something new from you."

"Come on, Carl. Let's go grab a beer. I'm buying."

They left as the Blackburn & Sons Funeral Home hearse was pulling into the back of the hospital. Bill cast a knowing nod toward the driver of Luanne's next ride. All in a day's work, thought Bill. All in a day's work.

The Department of Medical Allotment and Continuous Sustainability, or D-MACS, was a relatively new branch of the US Department of Health and Human Services. Working in tandem with the Centers for Medicare and Medicaid Services, the agency was created to address the government's mandate of health care for all. D-MACS was meant to systematically reduce the skyrocketing costs of healthcare. At the time, the United States ranked last in healthcare outcomes when compared to the top ten industrial nations worldwide. Yet, when it came to overall healthcare costs compared to other top-tier countries, they were strictly number one. Indeed, D-MACS was established to give the impression to the unsuspecting, non-clinical, ever-trusting public that the government was finally going to turn these statistics around. The agency was given over-reaching authority to address many healthcare issues, including access to care, clinical outcomes, administrative efficiency, and average cost per person.

Most of the press releases regarding D-MACS were well scripted and designed to divert the attention from the "real" money-slashing opportunities developed by the agency. For example, the much hyped 3.5 million dollars that were allocated for spreading awareness of the dangers of inactivity (remember the "Get Up and Move" campaign?) was paltry compared to the 1.2 billion dollars saved in actual Medicare payments, which was achieved through changes in eligibility (or some might say "ineligibility") for higher acuity healthcare. Thanks to panelists at D-MACS, not everyone was eligible for health care, as actuary tables ended up replacing PDRs on physicians' nightstands. A new era of healthcare had begun. Oh, sure, conspiracy theorists came awfully close to exposing the truth, but with the right amount of pressure on the right people, no one was ever the wiser. There was no turning back.

Healthcare would never be the same.

WHERE'D THE TIME GO?

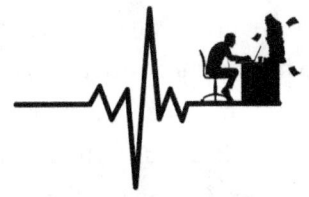

CHAPTER TWO

As the microwave slowly counted down to zero, Evan's soul faded just a little bit more. This wasn't the first time he sensed his purpose in life ebb toward hopelessness. When Jenna Thompson broke his heart in eighth grade by going to the Callaway Junior High Dance with Luke Redman instead of him, he first felt the pangs of "why me?" (Granted, Evan hadn't asked her or, well, hadn't ever actually spoken to her due to crush-induced paralysis.) When Evan finally found his voice and (imagined) confidence to audition for the eleventh grade high school "California Dreamin'" drama/musical and didn't even get selected as an alternate, the continued twinges of "what are you doing with your life" nudged at his soul again. But watching the Beef-N-Bean Burrito turn in the microwave, mocking him in its casual, carefree carousel rotations, Evan felt about as low as he had ever been. To be clear, it wasn't about the burrito. It was about something else. Something Evan hadn't taken the time to pursue.

Love.

Well, let's not kid ourselves. Evan's was not an atten-
tion-grabbing face in a crowd. Nor even in a non-crowd.
What was the opposite of "flashy"? Evan. Plain, nondescript. Always the friend. Evan's average mug was not lost
on him either. So he dove head-first into academics, finding
success in the classroom, especially math and science. Both
fields seemed to "get" Evan, and the feelings were mutual.
High school was a snap. College was even easier as he could
focus all of his attention on his education without the typical
distractions of dating, parties ... a social life.

This never bothered Evan as he never noticed how life
was speeding by around him. Until recently. His rapid rise
through the ranks at D-MACS had created quite a buzz. It
had come easy to him, memorizing every D-MACS code
and all of the statistics utilized to predict health outcomes
and determine healthcare feasibility for end-users. Career
success: number one with a bullet. Matters of the heart: on
life-support with no apparent chance of survival.

As Evan pondered the lack of love prospects in his life,
the *ding* of the microwave signaling the burrito was heated
snapped him out of his reverie.

Back at his desk, Evan spent his lunch navigating the newest proposed recommendations for cost-containment from
his employer. Usually not one to question the decisions made
by those above him, Evan stopped mid-bite upon reading the
latest recommended change to scoring. Code changes were
common enough to be considered part of the process. But
this one. This one was challenging for Evan to process.

Of course prior medical history weighed heavily in pre-
dicting future health care outcomes. Hypertension, cardiac

disease, diabetes—all were game changers in determining the likelihood of continued viability. This was different. D-MACS called it "Status Quotient."

As a panelist, his calculations for granting health care now would include the social status and what was called the "future global impact factor" of the patient. Married or single. Family or childless. Working in one of the fifty-three predetermined essential fields or in an outlier. The answers would impact future scores. For Evan, this took science out of the equation and injected something more sinister for him to consider: the subjective nature of *why* someone should be provided healthcare instead of the likelihood of healthcare success based on *scientific* studies. Evan dropped his half-eaten burrito in the trash and called the only person he could think of to discuss this issue. He'd know what to do.

Harry felt like he had the perfect job. He had grown up in the era of wizened barkeeps who would listen to the problems of their intoxicated patrons while they methodically wiped mahogany bars with a white towel. Some people were born talkers, with something to say to anyone who would listen. Others, like Harry, were born listeners. All his life, people shared pieces of their soul with Harry. And Harry was always glad to listen.

Only three obvious career choices existed for the Harrys of the world. Counselor, priest, or bartender. Professional counselors required an advanced education. For Harry, who got his high school diploma through the good graces of sympathetic teachers, this was not even a remote possibility.

To be a priest, well, such a job required believing in something more than what could be seen right in front of him. And Harry was not that imaginative. Keeping bar, however, while giving aspiring alcoholics someone to lament to—*that* was something he always knew he could do. And so he did. And for forty-two years, he could be counted on to mop up spilled drinks and freshly shed tears at Houlihan's Hideaway on 17th Street, six nights a week.

"So I says, 'I was just fine *before* I met you, and I'll be just fine *after* you're outta my hair." The story always started the same. And to be honest, most of 'em finished the same as well.

As the waterworks flowed, the story shifted from bravado to despair.

"WHY?!?!!? I gave that woman the best years of my life!"

Harry's towel deftly maneuvered around the lonely loser with surgical precision. He was equally as skilled in probing the inner recesses of his "patient's" thoughts and repressed memories. "Didn't you mention sleeping around with your secretary ... and your wife's sister?"

"OH, HERE WE GO!" exploded the imbibed lonely heart. "What on earth does that have to do with anything? I ... I ... OH NO, WHAT HAVE I DONE ..." etcetera, etcetera as the newly found single realized that maybe, possibly, inexplicably, he had a role in his own undoing.

The final count for the poor sot approached, and this one was rapidly headed for a Muhammad Ali quality KO. As his head hung low on his chest, muffled sobs of "Why? Why?" were sent up while Harry silently counted to ten, declaring the pathetic pugilist not only down for the count but also permanently retired from the sport.

As Harry continued his swift navigation of the bar with his towel, he looked up to see his nephew walk through the door.

Giving him a familiar nod, his brother's son trudged to the table in the back.

Evan sat down at the table nearest the kitchen in the back of the bar and waited for Harry. He had spent most of his childhood in the back of Houlihan's Hideaway. For many years, he'd show up after school, helping to clean, stock, sweep—menial tasks that helped him realize he did not want to *work*-work for a living. Too many calluses, too much sweat, and too much exhaustion.

But it wasn't all work during his formative years, watching his uncle tend bar. One summer, he had used empty vodka boxes to make an impenetrable fort in the pantry in the kitchen. He had lined it with a sleeping bag, and there, he began his first real love affair. Books. Shakespeare, Dickens, Tolstoy ... all the old, dead authors, sure. They had their place.

The reading he did during that impressionable summer he would never forget. Some fondly remembered the first time they crossed the seductive doorway from childhood to adulthood with a willing partner. Evan smilingly recalled his mistress with the same doe eyes and youthful yearnings. The Scarpetta novels by Patricia Cornwell. Oh, how they filled him with wonder and excitement and solidified his decision to somehow, someway be involved in the medical field. Maybe be a world-renowned cancer researcher. Possibly dabble in the realm of discovering a cure or two (did he dare go for three?) for terminal illnesses that had plagued the not-as-daring medical community over the years. The possibilities were endless! It was in the fort, in the dirty back pantry of Houlihan's Hideaway that Evan knew he would change the world. Dreams were good, no?

Harry startled Evan out of his reverie. "What's up, squirt?"

Evan never divulged personal struggles or inner demons to anyone other than his uncle. His dad was a great guy, don't be deceived. And his mom, well, moms were good for comfort foods and awkward hugs, and his was no different. Yet he never was able to let his guard down with either of them. Focused on the wrong things, you know? For instance, could anyone blame Evan for never being genuine with his folks again after being dumped by Sally Sheridan? At the fragile, impressionable age of seventeen, Evan poured his heart out to his father and mother over dinner. His dad chose to make jokes about Sally being "out of your league, kid," and his mom focused on Evan's need to accept his lot in life and stay in the "friend zone." He made a vow then and there to never again bring to them matters of the heart. And he kept his word.

"You seem like you got the world on your shoulders. What gives?" Harry gave his arm a nudge.

"What's up with the crying coot at the counter?"

Harry eyed the man with his head on the bar, now mumbling, "Why? Why?" in a tone slurred by alcohol and seeped in dawning realization.

"Problems with his old lady. Couldn't keep it in his pants, and she got tired of his philandering. Had it coming. He's done. I already set him up with three more Harvey Wallbangers, so we got some time. Tell me what's going on with you. Haven't seen you 'round here in a while."

Evan scrubbed his face. "Sorry about that. Work is gang-busters right now, and I haven't had a minute break."

"A man can only work so many hours in a day. Balance, kiddo, balance. If you were to die tomorrow ..."

"... would you have made the world a better place?" Evan finished for him. "I know, I know."

Harry had a lot of mantras. And sayings. And colloquial-isms. Seemed like Uncle Harry had a mildly relatable saying for just about anything put his way.

"Things are bad, Harry, really bad."

"Like my mama always said, "It's always darkest before the storm.""

"Hey Harry. I just lost my job."

"Well, to make an omelet, you gotta break a few eggs.

Actually, his comebacks never made much sense. However, his clientele never complained, especially after the third or fourth drink. Sometimes this was humorous, but often times it was confusing to the sober listener. Evan chose his words carefully. "I'm not sure what to do about my, uh, job right now. It's heading down a direction I don't like."

Now Uncle Harry had no idea what Evan did. He'd al-ways been vague in his descriptions, dangling words like government and health care and computers. Things of no interest to Harry. It was better that way. No one in his fam-ily knew his job was determining who received health care, essentially choosing who lived and who died. Had they known, there would have been some tough conversations. Evan wasn't into tough conversations.

"What direction is that?" Harry absently polished the

wooden tabletop with the flair of a maestro leading the symphony.

Evan tracked the cloth as it made hypnotizing swishes back and forth over the smooth surface. "I think I'm being asked to kill a lot more people."

The towel stopped mid-polish as Harry slowly looked at him as if for the first time. "I'm listening."

Evan regretted the words as soon as he'd spoken. Backtrack. Dodge and weave.

"Just kidding. It's just management is changing the rules midstream, and you know I'm not much for change."

Harry narrowed his eyes, and Evan did his best not to squirm. "Change can be good, y'know. As long as you know the who's and the what's and the why's. Have you talked with anyone about it at work?"

"Not yet. I just got the memo. Mandatory staff meeting about it tomorrow morning. With most work issues, I just sit, listen, make adjustments, and keep on keeping on. But this time, I dunno. I feel like I need to do something drastic. Something outrageous. I guess I'm—well, I ... I ... feel I'm at a crossroad, and I'm not sure what to do about it."

The towel resumed its polishing, and Harry's brow cleared. "Well, you've always been a smart kid. I know you will know the right thing to do. But if you want any advice ..." Harry drifted off as he tended to do at this point. He never forced suggestions on anyone, which Evan appreciated.

He needed more information before making any decisions so decided to retreat from the conversation. "Yeah, I should let this one simmer a bit. When I need direction, I know I can count on you, Harry."

"Anytime, kiddo. I gotta go prop up our sad sack over at the bar. Let me know how I can help. And don't be a stranger!"

As Evan got up from the table, Harry strolled back to his spot at the bar and caught the intoxicated fornicator moments before he hit the floor after downing all of the prescribed drinks. Another satisfied customer. Evan shook his head as he walked toward the door.

SQUARE PEG, ROUND HOLE

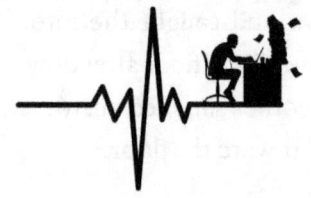

CHAPTER THREE

"It isn't that bad, is it?" In all actuality, it was.

"What if I brush it to the side a bit … like so … and … 'Voila!' That's better, right?" Wrong.

In the history of bad hair days, there had been three instances of traffic-stopping, stranger-gawking, "I-wish-I-could-unsee-what-I-just-saw" bad hair days in Peg's life. First was the fourth grade "I can trim my bangs myself" disaster. Next came the Big League Chew debacle, when she fell asleep with an *entire* bag in her mouth. No amount of peanut butter would get that out. And third was, of course, the "I'm ready for a new look" mistake at the local Kwik Kutz hair salon in which the stylist, unbeknownst to Peg, was ready to take out her frustrations of having her boyfriend run off with her best friend.

After giving herself her first ever at-home dye job (Sassy Summer Fun by Color-Rific) *and* a quick trim to rid herself of split ends, Peg looked like someone in need of a good hat. The results of her efforts left her in a sour mood.

"Good job, Peg. Way to go, Peg. It'll grow out, Peg." Peg's

efforts to self-remedy through positive thinking fell as flat as the orange strands crookedly hanging down her face.

"Hat time."

Fortunately (there you go, Peg! Way to see things positively!) the rainy afternoon made the rest of the city folks appear in need of a "do"-over as well. So Peg grabbed her laptop, tied a silk scarf over her hair, and headed to Cuppa Joe's around the corner to log in for work. She hoped it wasn't too busy—she wanted as little face-to-face time in line as possible.

The door jingled as she entered and the barista grinned, pointing at a steaming cup. "Got ya covered, Peg! Saw you coming. Caramel frappe with skim milk and cinnamon, right?" the barista called to Peg as she entered the shop.

She sheepishly gave a nod. "Thanks, Jeffrey. How'd you ever guess?" Grabbing the frappe, she wondered how she would ever be able to let him know that she had tired of the caramel frappe concoction several weeks ago. But he was so nice. And Peg was so non-confrontational. And ... well, if someone did something nice for you, you just focused on that, right? But ... oh, how good the cocoa-cabana coffee looked in the poster on the door.

Last Tuesday, she tried to change it up, and Jeffrey had laughed and said, "Good one, Peg! You almost got me! Here's your usual!" as he slid her *another* caramel frappe.

Peg took her usual place (and usual beverage), where she plugged in her laptop. As it booted up, she sipped on the beverage.

"Today I seize the day. Today is mine to conquer. Today is ..." Peg ran through the self-motivating phrases her therapist had recommended to her.

But she wasn't feeling it. *What is it, Peg? The hair? The dreary weather? The same-old, same-old coffee? What is it?* Her gaze wandered to a D-MACS job poster pinned to the bulletin board surrounded by want-ads, sub-let ads, and "Learn to Play GUITAR in six easy lessons!" ads. It wasn't the first time she'd read the poster. For several days, it had drawn her attention. Something about the Uncle Sam caricature pointing at her and the red-white-and-blue "We Need YOU" lettering in the bubble over his top hat.

It was Sam's wry smile, she admitted. So knowing. So inviting. The slight upturn of his lips seemed to say, "Yes … it's you, Peg! This is the opportunity you've been waiting for!"

And she *was* wanting a change. She wasn't *totally* miserable working the other end of the InstaChat assistant line for the largest nationwide auto insurance company around.

"Hi! I'm Peg, your virtual assistant."

"Yes, we cover all customers, regardless of driving records."

"I'll be glad to have an agent call you."

Boring.

Peg decided then and there to go against her instincts and not talk herself out of applying for a new job. *I mean, it's a job with the government, so it's got to be a great opportunity, right? Secure benefits. Clear direction. Helping out one's fellow citizens. How great is that?*

After about fifteen minutes of answering some seemingly unconnected questions, Peg was second guessing her decision. The answers could range from "Strongly Disagree" to "Strongly Agree".

"I enjoy helping people." Sure.

"I am a quick learner." Definitely.

"I can make definitive decisions." Ummm ... well ... sometimes, maybe.

"Healthcare is a privilege, not a choice." Wait ... what?

"I enjoy being a part of a team." OK, sure.

"Our society would benefit from enforcing better health-care choices." What does that mean?

"People should have a limit to how much healthcare they are given based on predictive factors." Huh?

Peg reached out to close her laptop and scrap the whole carpe diem baloney and delete her partially completed application when Uncle Sam decided at that moment to intently stare directly into her soul.

"Stop overthinking everything, Peg," she thought. "It's a government job. The government is there to help people. You are reading way too much into the questions. It's a computer job for D-MACS. Period."

Peg finished the questionnaire, uploaded her resumé to the portal, and hit "Enter". She had not felt this emboldened in years. Or scared. She should have listened to her instincts. Peg's life was about to change, she felt it. Exactly how was beyond her limited imagination.

"The government is there to help people." Good one, Peg.

The Department of Medical Allotment and Continuous Sustainability received approximately twelve hundred applications per month for various positions. Use of the Likert scale had streamlined the ability of Human Resources to sort out applicants and ensure the appropriate departments received vetted respondents. Of the twelve hundred applications, roughly four hundred were immediately sent a standard response email: "We have received your application. Thank you for your interest in D-MACS. Unfortunately, we have selected a more qualified candidate for the position. Have a nice day." Another three hundred were forwarded to other governmental agencies for consideration. And about two hundred were deleted immediately based on the respondent's inability to correctly follow the application process.

The remaining three hundred applicants were sent to the appropriate subsection of D-MACS for review. Of those three hundred, only a handful were sent to Evan's department. Those that met the preferred profile as determined by the online application process were followed up by a phone call to ensure the qualifications were in alignment with D-MACS expectations. It was an arduous process and, of those who received a phone call, usually only one or two candidates made the final cut for an in-person interview.

Richard Brannigan received Peg's application and reviewed her answers over a mediocre cup of Douwe Egbert instant coffee. Each month, he received applications for review and very few received a phone call. However, Peg's answers intrigued him.

"Either 'Peg' is an automated Russian computer bot that has figured out the D-MACS code for candidate selection ... or she is the most perfect respondent I've seen in quite a while," Richard mused over sips of his lukewarm beverage. Richard was feeling pressure from his superiors to fill vacant positions, and that could sometimes skew your perception.

Richard had been one of the hiring and recruitment

managers for D-MACS for the past seven years. The prior three years were spent sweating it out on the panel with abysmal results. He never quite grasped the nuances required for the position. So many damn diseases and medical conditions. Who the hell could keep up with them all? If not for the insight and foresight of the medical review team to have multiple members on the decision-making panel at all times, Richard would have single-handedly wiped out enough patients to fill Wrigley Field. Just when he thought he had it, another case would come along that would prompt Richard to toss them in the reject pile.

"Hey, uh, Rich ..." Richard could still hear his panel supervisor's patronizing tone ... and smell his penchant for Cool Ranch Doritos breathing down his neck. "Can we talk about Ms. Culver?"

"Yeah, sure ... whatever. What about her?"

"So. Ms. Culver. Remember her chart? Thirty-one-year-old. History of a tonsillectomy and not much else? Came in with clear cut appendicitis?"

"I ... maybe ... not sure ... why?"

"Well, she scored a seven per the program actuary, and she averaged a six point eight among the other members of the panel."

"So?"

"You scored her a seventy-seven! I mean, Jesus, Richard! I didn't think our review scores even went that high! What the hell were you thinking?"

"Well ... uh I remember—oh, wait, that wasn't her ... Oh yeah, she was the one I suspected of faking symptoms and—no ... that wasn't her either. What are you saying?"

"I'm saying you stink at this. This isn't your cup of tea. We put you through extra training, gave you additional orientation, even paired you with Reggie, Margo, and Juan. It just isn't working out. However, an opening in another department might be up your alley. What do you know about recruitment?"

Seven years later, Richard held onto the best application to come across his desk in years. Richard dialed the provided mobile number and cleared his throat to deliver what he hoped would be the smoothest recruitment phone call Peg had ever received.

Those who can't, well, they teach, right? And those who can't teach … they work in HR.

OLD DOGS, NEW TRICKS

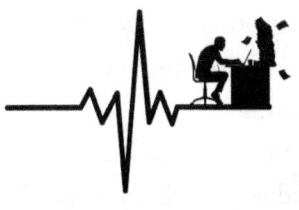

CHAPTER FOUR

Adelman's Bakery was *the* place for the best bialys. Any schmuck could order a bagel and ruin it with an inch-thick layer of cream cheese or (Oy vey!) peanut butter. Ms. Horowitz could vividly recall the moment thirty-five years ago that she saw this culinary atrocity at Schuler's in New York City. Like any self-respecting person should, she walked straight up to the man who was about to stab his teeth into the blasphemous peanut concoction and slapped it out of his hand, sending it sailing across the coffee shop. She cracked a crooked smile, remembering how the bagel sailed through the air and stuck, peanut butter side first, to the store's window, like a cautionary message to anyone else who tried this affront to Jewish baked goods. A proud moment in the Horowitz legacy for sure!

But bagels were not the planned purchase this morning. Bialys at Adelman's were as good as they came for many gourmands within a twenty-block radius. Ms. Horowitz had a pint-sized tub of tuna salad (from Kravitz's Deli, of course) in her refrigerator that was simply waiting to be piled high on one of Adelman's finest. This was worth the walk.

Ms. Horowitz made the three-block trek to Adelman's like clockwork every other day. Normally she kept a scowl on her face to ward off any potential well-wishers.

"How are you today?"

"Old and constipated, who wants to know?"

"Lovely day today, wouldn't you say?"

"If I liked smog, the smell of day-old wino's piss, and your halitosis, I guess I would. Other than that, screw you."

Ms. Horowitz was not one for thoughtless pleasantries. But today, oh, today … Was something special in the air today? Had anything specific happened? Social Security check came in the mail yesterday. Well, yeah. The house cleaner didn't ruin the carpet for once. Surprising, yes, but not very mood elevating, one would say. What in the world … got it!

Ms. Horowitz laughed out loud as she recalled the conversation she had with her nitwit sister. Her sister and her equally airheaded husband. Oy vey! How they could drive a sane person to the nuthouse! But yesterday … yesterday was a masterpiece if she had to say so herself. Maya was going on and on and on about her art class or her kids or her chronic arthritis or the way Levi devoured her inedible cooking, when Ms. Horowitz interrupted the ramblings.

"You know, I'm the reason why Nonna never liked you."

Maya paused. "Um, what did you say?"

"Nonna She never liked you. Always liked me best."

In a choked voice, Maya stuttered, "What do you mean?"

Ms. Horowitz held back a cackle. "You want to know why?"

The silence on the other end of the line peppered with an occasional sniffle was all the confirmation she needed. "Remember her prized crystal wine decanter? I told her you chipped it."

"You ... you ... what? That wasn't me!"

"I know it wasn't you, nimwit. But I couldn't have told her it was me. I mean, it *was* somewhat your fault since you dodged out of the way when I threw the shoe at your head. Anyway, I told her that night and swore that you didn't mean to chip her decanter, but, you know, you were so careless and clumsy ..."

The silence on the phone and then the palpable heat emanating through the receiver was priceless. The way she finally shut up her sister after keeping the secret for sixty-five years was simply too wonderful to fully digest. The amazing satisfaction of spilling the beans combined with the sight of Adelman's Bakery straight ahead was glorious. The morning sun shining upon her made her squint and she smiled for the first time in months. Surely that is what kept her from noticing until too late the speeding taxi that ran into her and knocked her off her feet. She flew a good thirty feet into the display window of Thompson's Fine China and Glassware. The crystal decanter that fell from its shelf, embedding jagged shards into her hands, arms, chest, and face, didn't kill her. It only made the midah k'neged midah that much more cosmic. Oy vey ...

As the ambulance pulled into the emergency department entrance, the face sheet with clinical overview and demographics for Noa Horowitz, a seventy-two-year-old Caucasian female, pedestrian vs. car, had been already sent to D-MACS with the panel decision being determined even before the vehicle came to a stop. The EMTs were instructed by the ED triage to bring the stretcher to Trauma Bay 3 for treatment. Terrell Shaver had been with County Dispatch Ambulance Service for almost twenty-three years. Being in the same dispatch unit for so long had its pros and cons. Pros? He knew which drive-thru burger joints used fresh meat on Tuesdays (Burger Buddy's on 39th) and which drive-thru sandwich shops re-used day-old meats three days in a row (Flint's Sandwich Shoppe on 10th—actually, it's probably best to never go to Flint's Sandwich Shoppe on 10th any day of the week, to be honest). Cons? The damn changes to protocols and procedures at D-MACS. *I mean. Damn! Do you want me to bring in patients to get help or not?* Seemed like every other week there was a new mandate from D-MACs that didn't seem to make sense. Take this old bird who got mowed down by a taxicab in front of the Jewish deli downtown. When Terrell started with County Dispatch, the old lady would have been taken to the closest hospital due to her injuries. Nowadays? The panel had to dictate where to send patients, meaning sometimes they sat at the scene, waiting to know which way to go. Sending this lady to Regional General added fifteen minutes to her transport, decreasing her chance of making it. If you were to ask Terrell though … maybe that's what D-MACS was trying to do. Damn!

Murray slammed his fist down on the desk in his cubicle, shaking the computer screens of those around him.

"Seriously? A mandatory half-day training session on Status Quotient? Uh-uh. No freakin' way. Evan, did you see this crap?"

Evan did see the memo and was relieved it had been scheduled. Surely D-MACS would spend this time explaining how the panel was *NOT* actually going to weigh their scores on a new scale, taking subjective data into account to screen for health care availability. Did Murray have the same concerns about this direction as he did?

"I did, Murr. It's crazy, right? We can't change up scores based on whether or not a person is giving back to society, or something like that, right?"

"Who the F cares, Evan? I already do that, anyway. Don't you? These old geezers think they got an ice cube's chance in Hades to qualify for open heart surgery? They're about to kick it anyway. I'm talking about management thinking I'm rescheduling my date for some bogus update on our scoring metrics.

"Oh yeah. I mean ... sure ... Rita sounds like a great reason to skip out on this."

"Rita? Not that wacko. I dumped her midway through our last date. 'Want some gum, Murray?' 'Have you tried this new breath mint, Murray?' 'I love my dentist, Murray. I go every six months. What about you, Murray?' Good grief. What a head case. When she went to the restroom, I skedaddled outta there. Who needs that kind of aggravation, right?"

Evan mentally applauded Rita's attempt to steer Murray into the newly discovered world of dental health.

"I'm meeting Tabitha for early drinks and dinner. Met her on the Lovestar app. Instant connection. She might be the one. Can you cover for me and take notes?"

"Sure, Murr. It'll probably just be some bureaucratic spiel anyways. Enjoy yourself."

"I always do!"

The auditorium was two-thirds full when Evan made his way to an empty seat.

Richard stopped him as he edged by. "Oh, hey, Evan—I was going to reach out to you this afternoon—glad I saw you here. I found a replacement for Carla, and I was thinking you would be the perfect panelist to onboard her. She starts next week. Peg Something-or-Other. I'll send you her resumé when I get back to my desk. Thanks, sport." He released his death grip on Evan's arm, signaling he was done with the conversation.

"Um, I don't know, Rich. I mean, jeez, isn't it Murray's turn to orient a new hire? I'm figuring out this new process that corporate is pushing on us and, well, Murray's not a bad panelist himself ..."

"Actually, Murray *is* up to onboard the next hire but ... you know ... I mean, c'mon Evan. This new hire. Peg. She's, well ... she's *female*. The, uh, higher ups thought after the complaints from Keisha, Joanna, Tina, and Charlene ... well, it would be easier for everyone if he only oriented guys. You know what I mean?"

"Sure, Richard. I guess so. Send me her info, and I'll do it. Can you also send me the checklist again so I can document the next steps with her?" Evan had heard about the complaints regarding Murray but hadn't known HR was aware as well.

"You got it, pal. Thanks!"

Evan continued down the aisle and found a seat just as the D-MACS admin team was dimming the lights and getting the PowerPoint presentation up on the screen.

"Everyone, please take a seat. We're having a slight bit of technical difficulty. Um, Ellen, can you help with this?"

As Ellen, the executive assistant to the medical director of D-MACS, fumbled with input sources and logins, the rest of the D-MACS coders and panelists found seats and quietly talked among themselves about their thoughts on Status Quotient and what it actually meant.

"They're trying to reduce hospitalizations since inpatient numbers nationwide were still over budget."

"Nah, I heard they're trying to covertly control the population through increased mortality rates."

"Well, D-MACS was being secretly controlled by the Dark State."

"Wait, I thought this was a meeting about changing the menu items in the cafeteria. Am I in the wrong place?"

The lights dimmed and the PowerPoint showed brightly on the auditorium's large screen.

D-MACS
Director Dr. Harold Thompkins, MD, MBA, CPA, CITP
Providing New Avant Guard Improvements to Healthcare Affordability for ALL!
Beta Test Site Utilization and Implementation
When Dr. Thompkins cleared his throat, the room fell

quiet. "Thank you all for coming on such short notice. Ellen, thank you for getting the presentation up. OK, so everyone knows why we're here. So let's jump right in. I don't have to tell you how important our role is here at D-MACS. I mean, as a doctor for thirty-seven years, I've seen some changes in my time. Why, it seems like yesterday I was doing my residency at the Medical Center in Cleveland. One time ..."

For fifteen minutes, Dr. Thompkins droned on about "in my day" and "we sure had it tough" stories that had been regaled to all numerous times before. For many, it was the seventh or eighth time of hearing about delivering a baby in the back of a Mitsubishi Galant on the side of I-90 at three in the morning. while a frigid Lake Erie brought in record amounts of snow, wait, was it snow? Maybe it was sleet. Maybe it was some sleet, some rain, some snow. Well, dang. What was it? Who could really tell? One thing for sure, he and Steve Levy, wait ... was it Steve or Shane? Half the room dozed until the valiant doctor of old finally segued into the purpose of the meeting.

"As you see, the next logical step for D-MACS is to ensure that healthcare is available for those who would benefit most from it. This is where each of you comes in to play at this vital time. As the beta test site for the newest initiative, we are the pioneers for the future of healthcare. Each of you has been tasked to be the ones to determine if Status Quotient is a part of said future. Let's look at it a bit closer, shall we?"

Evan listened with rapt attention as Dr. Thompkins explained how Status Quotient was developed over the course of the past several months through utilizing AI to delineate which patients not only had the most likely chance of full recovery from various diseases, illnesses, and calamities but which ones would actually be of benefit to pushing the next wave of healthcare sustainability into the future.

"As a physician who provides input and makes decisions for D-MACS, I still rely on the four principles I vowed to uphold when I became a new MD all those years ago: that of beneficence, non-maleficence, justice, and respect for our patient's autonomy. In the healthcare environment of today, doing what is in the best interest of our patients is more important than ever. We must ensure we can fiscally help the ever-expanding number of patients covered under D-MACS policy. And this is where Status Quotient really was born and where each of you fit in. YOU get to be a part of the exciting world of improving healthcare affordability for all!"

The next few slides Dr. Thompkins reviewed were worse than Evan expected, leaving him more confused.

"Let's see ...that's two old fashions, one martini—extra dirty—and a gin and tonic, right?" Harry announced as he placed the four drinks on the table for the two couples.

"Ooh, Ben! Look at this! This must be a martini! I feel just like James Bond!" Quickly changing her delight into what Harry could only assume was supposed to be intense seriousness, she sternly asked Harry, "It's shaken, not stirred, right?"

Harry confirmed to the novice inebriate that her well-brand martini (which was mostly olive juice and garnish) was created *exactly* how the British spy would have insisted.

Walking back to his station behind the bar, Harry attempted to calculate how many times he had heard that joke over his career when Evan came through the door and took a seat near the back. Harry nodded in acknowledgement as he finished his rounds on the smattering of customers before joining him at his table.

"If your face were a street sign, it would say, 'Danger: Road Out Ahead'. What's the trouble?"

Evan always appreciated Harry's ability to size him up and go straight to the main issue without small talk. He shoved his hand through his hair. "I dunno, Harry. Work just told me to do things that don't mesh with my beliefs. Am I being too sensitive? I just dunno."

"A man that sacrifices his beliefs, is like a broken compass. He'll simply wander aimlessly with no way of knowing his true North."

Evan *almost* always appreciated Harry's ability to offer up thought-provoking idioms. Almost always.

"Listen, squirt. I have heard a million and a half stories over the years from a million and a half sad sots. But you? You ain't like them. I can tell from your expression you already know the right thing to do."

Evan *never* appreciated Harry's ability to never tell him what to do while, at the same time, telling him exactly what to do.

"I know, Harry." He huffed out a breath. "Except this isn't like anything I've ever experienced before. I seriously have no idea what the next step should be. And while I'm not against change and progress and such, if something's working, why break it? It's counterintuitive to everything I know." He'd been asked to do a lot during his time there. Yet this remained beyond his ability to rationalize. He focused on his hands on the tabletop. "A part of me just wants to go along with it."

Harry made an unintelligible noise in the back of his throat.

Evan swung his gaze to his face." Don't get me wrong. I'm thinking about actually questioning authority, here, which you know isn't my thing, right? And if I go against this new requirement, it's probable I'll face consequences— maybe even retaliation. I don't even know where to start. I mean, I guess I could— nah, that wouldn't work. Or would it?" Evan fell quiet, imagining a scenario in which he addressed his demons head on. He was in a daydream for a few moments before he felt Harry's gaze.

Harry studied him with the same mesmerizing intensity that Kaa used on Mowgli in the *Jungle Book*. Harry rarely used his hypnotizing stare on him. In fact, the last time he did, Evan ended up trying out for the seventh-grade basketball team (at a whopping four feet two inches tall) and actually making it. Evan *hated* that stare. Look away, Evan! Look away!

Too late. He was done for. "You can stop with the stare tactic, Harry. I got it." Evan heaved another sigh. Harry's lips quirked as he polished the table with his towel, laboring with increased energy, a fact that did not go unnoticed by Evan, who couldn't help squirming in his own awkward silence.

Finally, Evan caved and shared what was on his mind.

"I guess I was hoping I wasn't right. Does that make any sense?"

"Perfect sense. Someone once said, 'The hardest thing in life is knowing which bridges to cross and which to burn.' But I know you, and I know your heart. You got this."

Harry stood and moved toward his post at the bar when Evan got up and gave him an earnest hug. He didn't typically show affection, but Harry had helped him navigate his confused thoughts. It felt right to show appreciation.

Harry gave a quick hug in return, with a couple of obligatory back pats. "It's gonna be OK, squirt. Trust yourself."Evan didn't let go. If anything, he might have held in a sniffle.

"C'mon, Evan." Harry shifted like he was going to back away, but instead, he gathered Evan in even closer and murmured some "there, there's" above his head.

Evan, basking in this moment of comfort accidentally made eye contact with some bar patrons staring daggers at their apparently unwelcome display of support. Breaking the hug, Evan wiped the tears from his eyes and complained about how the dust in Harry's bar was causing his allergies to flare. Then he ducked out of the bar, leaving Harry to resume his duties as the patron saint of potable poisons. In fact—Evan snorted—Harry was Houlihan's version of His Holiness himself, minus the funny hat. He was probably blessing each inebriated soul in attendance as he resumed his pouring out of communion—sans the stale wafers.

SMOKE AND MIRRORS

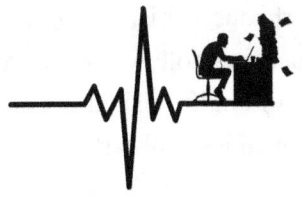

CHAPTER FIVE

Sharon McAllister sensed something was amiss. She had been awakened several times from her slumber in her recliner with wicked indigestion. That, in of itself, was not so unusual. Having resigned herself to sleeping in her Barcalounger a little over a year ago to assist with her sleep apnea and acid reflux, she knew what heartburn felt like. Hell yeah, she'd had some wicked heartburn in her time. A sly smile crept upon her round face as she thought about the night just last Wednesday in which she had gotten Chuck Truck delivered. A slab of BBQ ribs. A quart of slaw. A quart of baked beans. A pint (diet secret!) of Brunswick stew. And chocolate pie. Oh! The pie. And, boy howdy, did she pay for it that night. Every hour, on the hour, she was awakened with radiating pain across her chest, up to her neck, and down her arms. Worth it!

But this pain was different. No matter how she tried, it wasn't going away. TUMS didn't touch it. Rolaids was no good.

Sharon had fallen asleep the other night watching "Grey's Anatomy" reruns, and hadn't a patient come in with a heart attack? And didn't she say it was a different pain than usual heartburn? Dammit. Sharon picked up the phone and dialed 9-1-1.

"If I make it through this, I'm gonna get in shape. I swear!" Sharon made her hollow, empty promise to the scattered pizza boxes and half-finished Mountain Dew bottles crowding her coffee table. "I swear!"

"So did HR get you your badge, parking decal, and direct deposits situated?" Evan asked, trying to place himself between Peg and Murray. The jerk was making tremendous efforts to get the gold medal in the Olympic event of leering and ogling. At his current pace, he was an odds-on favorite to win it all. Evan wanted to kick him in the shins.

Peg nodded. She seemed the quiet type, though the way her eyes darted back to Murray, Evan figured first-day jitters weren't the only reason she was nervous.

Evan decided to move the onboarding review to the department's conference room, away from Murr's voyeuristic tendencies. The room was set up by D-MACS to provide space for small meetings, in-services, consultations, and any multi-use needs. The glass walls situated in the middle of the large room allowed for visibility and accountability while at the same time giving some respite from prying eyes.

As with most government agencies, many workers were tasked to add various roles to their job descriptions. Notoriously slow, many functions of Human Resources were delegated to others to increase some semblance of efficiency. Evan was given access years ago to add new users to the panelists roster, and he quickly got Peg entered into the database. Once he had given her access, he pulled up several different learning modules and spreadsheets on the multiple computer screens while Peg watched. As different monitors lit up various tables and medical definitions, Evan continued with his orientation.

"So, you see, the end game here is to provide a score for the medical nuances each subject has in order for the most appropriate care to be given based on an aggregate score among several reviewers."

Blank stare.

Sensing Peg's overwhelm, Evan switched gears. "I think it would make more sense to walk through one together to get a sense of what you'll eventually be doing on your own. Sound good? Let's take this one for example."

Peg gave a nod.

As the patient's chart illuminated on the large computer monitor located in front of them, Evan narrated as he pointed out corresponding information on the screen.

"Let's see, seventy-one-year-old Caucasian female. Presented with vague substernal pain and epigastric discomfort. Mild nausea and vomiting. History includes fifty-five pack per year smoker, moderate alcohol consumption, Type 2 Diabetes, BMI indicates morbid obesity thanks to her 5'4" height and 245 pounds weight, hypercholesterolemia, hypertension ... this is classic, Peg. Classic." He turned to her. Same glazed eyes.

She bit her lip. "I'm not sure what to make of any of this. How do you know what all these words are? I mean, what is 'epigastric'? What is 'hypercholesterolemia'? I mean, what do I do with this?"

Evan flashed a smile of commiseration. He remembered those early days. "Well, I know these words are new to you, but if you scroll the cursor over any of them … like so … you can right click and get a definition. See? 'Epigastric' is the upper part of your abdomen. If you … yeah, you got it."

Peg took control of the computer mouse and right-clicked on various words, seeing how it worked.

"Once you do a few of these, you'll notice the same words over and over and over until you get a feel for the picture being painted in the chart. Yeah, you're getting it!"

Peg scrolled some, then cocked her head. "So, this lady is overweight with several health care problems. Smokes. Drinks. High cholesterol. Diabetes. High blood pressure. OK. So now what? I mean, what am I supposed to do with this?"

Sharon only had to wait about ten minutes for the ambulance to arrive. The EMTs who came to her small one-bedroom apartment made little to no effort to hide their contempt for her housekeeping skills and physical condition. Having gone on disability several years ago due to her chronic back pain, Sharon had essentially given up on any non-essential rituals like vacuuming and acts of daily hygiene. The EMTs got her vitals, required information, ran an EKG, which was scanned and uploaded to the system, and assisted her onto the stretcher.

The morphine administered for her complaints of chest pain was working, and she felt a sense of mellowness she'd never experienced before. "This ain't so bad," Sharon thought as she was transported out the front door and taken to the ambulance. She vaguely heard the EMTs talking as she drifted out of consciousness.

"I'm telling you, Terrell, ain't no way we're going to Regional with *this* one." The EMT nodded his head toward Sharon as he pushed the stretcher down the walkway to the truck. "I'd put a solid twenty on that, I mean solid."

"Easy money, Carlos. I'll take your bet."

They loaded her into the back of the ambulance and called it into Central Dispatch.

"Yeah, Dispatch, this is Shaver. We got a seventy-one-year-old obese female in need of cardiac assistance. She has responded well to morphine. Vitals are within normal limits. EKG? Yep— we sent it in. NSTEMI on the monitor. She's a big 'un. Nasal cannula two liters. Eighteen gauge IV in her left AC. We are dripping in some fluids. Where do you want us to take her?"

Sharon heard bits and pieces of the conversation between the EMTs and somebody and finally succumbed to a morphine sleep, thinking, "I'm in good hands. I'm gonna be OK. I'm gonna be OK ..."

Evan took control of the computer mouse and clicked on a tab that took them to the rating grid. "See right here? "This patient has been picked up by EMTs and is requesting direction on which hospital to take her to. So if you use her score of fifty-seven from her problem list and ... look ... see? The rating grid on this page shows you how to direct them according to current D-MACS algorithms. Once you get a handle of this, you won't really need to reference the tab as it'll be second nature to you. So she's being sent to an outlying hospital instead of the closest one, as her co-morbidities prohibit rapid resuscitative efforts. I mean, she's a fifty-seven, after all.

"Wait, what? I'm not sure I understand what it is we're doing here. We determine what type of health care she gets? Seems a bit backward. Doesn't the doctor know what's best? Shouldn't she go to the closest hospital and have a doctor give her every fighting chance?"

"Great question, Peg. You're *kinda* right in that the physician is still the most qualified to determine what would be the ideal plan of care for a patient. In a perfect world. But we aren't living in a perfect world. We are in D-MACS world. And that world looks at a bigger picture for the health of many versus the needs of one."

"That's terrible! Right? I mean, what do you mean 'ideal world'? Are you saying our job is to give a thumbs up or thumbs down to people's lives?"

Evan had seen this emotional realization and panic several times in numerous new hires over the years ... but Peg seemed to get it much, much faster than previous orientees. It was a pivotal moment for any new employee when they sensed they were on some sort of Death Panel. This would require calm and clarity to avoid losing Peg. And Peg seemed like she was going to be a good one ... making the next steps all the more crucial.

"Okay. Think of it this way. You have an entire stadium of people attending a ball game. Beautiful day. Mid-seventies. Couple of lazy clouds floating by without a care in the world.

Suddenly a catastrophic event occurs. I don't know. Maybe an earthquake. Maybe a fire. I don't know. But something big. So the folks in the know have to start triaging people to save the most lives. Who gets the needed help first? There are only so many that can be taken care of first—meaning some are assisted second, third, and so on. So who would you pick?"

"Well ... I mean this is a terrible thing to say, I guess, but wouldn't you start with the kids? Children first?"

"Great choice. Sure. So we round up all the kids first and get them rapid treatment. Why did you pick them, Peg? I mean, you're correct that in this scenario, those under eighteen years old would get a higher prioritization. But why exactly did you pick them?"

"I don't know. I mean, they're kids. They're the most vulnerable, and they're our future and all that. Right?"

"Okay, I see where you're going. Children are the future and whatnot. What about their chances of recovery though? What do you think about that?"

"Well, I guess children are by and large healthier and would bounce back from something better." The fog rapidly dissipated from her eyes.

This one was quick. "Yes, yes, they definitely would bounce back fast. But you said they would bounce back from something 'better.' Better than what, Peg?"

Peg was getting it. "Better than someone really old or someone with multiple health problems?"

"Bingo was his name-o. Exactly. Which is all we are doing here. Helping to ensure that those who are most likely to recover from whatever happens are able to rapidly get the treatments and plans without delay."

"So, what about those who are not in such good shape? What about this one on our screen, here?"

The EMTs received their orders to transport Sharon to the outlying facility on the north side of the city, bypassing several of the bigger healthcare centers on the way. Carlos laid a twenty-dollar bill on the dashboard of the ambulance and sulked. Having their dispatch urgency relegated to a level two, they drove the speed limit in the right-hand lane and turned off the lights and siren. Sharon's sonorous breathing resonated through the rig. The two EMT's knew from experience that, one: the morphine would keep her knocked out for at least another half hour. Two: plenty of time remained to hit a drive-through on the way to the hospital. And three: this patient was never going to return to home. It was amazing how fast they had assimilated to the relatively new world order for patient transport. Back in the day, they would have been reprimanded for not breaking the speed limit to drop off patients as fast as they could. Now? Stress level was reduced to a solid zero, as they were—more often than not—instructed to take their time in moving patients around the city. As they pulled into the drive-thru lane, they both smiled.

"Welcome to Wally's, whataya have? Wanna super-size that?"

Terrell and Carlos were in complete agreement. They definitely super-sized that.

Driving home, Peg smiled. For the first time in who knows how long, she felt like she was in the right place. I mean, sure, there was going to be a learning curve. But Evan said she was doing well and was even ahead of many new hires he had trained before. Plus, it was interesting work.

"I'm actually helping people!" she yelled out loud. Could it be possible this was the job for her? Other than stumbling over some of the medical terminology, she actually understood the premise. She caught a glimpse of herself in the rearview mirror and saw the hope in her eyes and the smile on her face and felt good about the day. "You did it, girl!" she encouraged the reflection in the mirror. "You did it!"

Driving home, Evan smiled. For the first time in who knew how long, he felt something he hadn't felt in a long time. Happy. Encouraged. Like he was in the right place. I mean, sure, Peg had a long way to go before she was ready to be a panelist on her own, but she was smart. She asked all the right questions and seemed to get it. They were able to go through several more charts before he had her check off some required computer-based learning. As Evan looked in the rearview mirror before changing lanes, he caught a glimpse of himself and saw a brightness in his eyes and a smile on his face he hadn't seen in quite a while and felt good about the day. "Good job!" he encouraged himself and made the decision to head to his uncle's bar to tell him the news. "Good job!"

"These numbers can't be right!" Earl Yarborough shouted into the phone. As CEO of D-MACS, Earl had earned a reputation for getting to the heart of financial reports and anticipating anything that came his way. With the most recent cuts to the budget by congress, he was confident the second quarter financial reports would positively reflect the changes he had mandated at D-MACS to get things in line. "GET YOUR BUTTS IN HERE NOW!" he yelled with spittle flying across the desk as he slammed down the phone. Loosening his tie and unbuttoning his collar, Earl slumped back in his desk chair and rubbed his eyes. "I'm too old for this" he mumbled as financial accountants and various bean counters hurried into the room, visibly shaken. They cowered together as if to brace for the verbal storm he was about to let loose their way.

Earl started his career in Chicago decades ago, working his way through various industries and just about every job title known to man. Car dealerships. Factory line foreman. Contractor. Poultry Plant Supervisor. Some might claim Earl couldn't commit to a job. But Earl would disagree. He would say (and he did in his autobiography *A Man for All Seasons*) that he was laser focused on one thing and one thing only: could he add something to the job that hadn't been done before? And no one could argue with his success. His seemingly meteoric rise to the top of D-MACS was not an easy feat, and Earl would be the first to tell you (as he did in his follow-up autobiography *To Err Is Human—but I Ain't Human!*) that his mantra, "results—not excuses," had carried him far. And it was this life motto, which he had made into a banner-sized sign hanging behind him in his office, that he pointed to as he addressed the financial group cowering before him.

"Tommy, what does that sign say? Huh? What. Does. It. SAY!?!?!?!?"

"Results—not excuses, sir."

"WHAT?!?!?! I can't hear you over the sniffling and mumbling!"

"I said, 'results—not excuses,' sir," Tommy said, louder.

"Good. You can read. But I didn't hire any of you to read, now did I? I hired you math geeks to help me look good with the numbers. And right now, when I check these financial reports, I ... don't ... *look* ... good, now do I?"

The assembled accountants quietly agreed with their CEO.

"No, sir."

"Not really."

"Well, perhaps there is a silver lining."

"Definitely not, sir."

Earl considered the one non-sycophant in the crowd. "What was that? Who said that? Was it you, Jan?"

"Um, no sir. It was me. Samantha. Samantha McAllister, sir."

Jan and the others silently, as if on cue, took half a step back, putting Samantha more clearly in his cross-hairs.

"OK, OK. Samantha McAllister. Oh yes, the Status Quotient ideator. Enlighten me. What in these reports do *you* see that these nimrods haven't seen?"

Samantha was the newest addition to the D-MACS administrative team. Having spent three years in DC as a congressional intern, she would have learned from the best on how to make data say anything you wanted. It was just a matter of how you looked at it. Earl needed that insight.

"If I may, sir?" Samanatha reached out for the reports Earl had been waving in their faces.

Earl, stunned by the boldness and brashness of this new-bie, slowly handed the stack of papers over.

Samantha quickly flipped through the report. "So in my review ... let's see ... ah, yes ... here it is, on page seven-teen. In my review of these reports, I noticed what could be the start of a positive narrative for the newest initiatives at D-MACS with our newest beta test site. See, sir ... here. When comparing cost escalation trends on page seventeen with the actual utilization trends of services to hospitals, physician practices, etc. on ... yes, here, on page twenty-four. You see the dramatic shift that our newest initiatives, as sub-tle as they may well be, are actually showing a positive trend when it comes down to the bottom line. I mean, after all, sir, I don't have to tell you how important Status Quotient could be for the entire D-MACS world, do I?"

Earl schooled his features so he wouldn't take on the gaping fish faces of the others. He didn't have any idea how important the beta test site could be. And apparently neither did the rest of them.

"On the one hand, costs have gone up—yes. That's to be expected due to the cost of running business. Our pay-ments for imaging studies, CT scans, X-rays, for example, are higher due to the higher utilization of procedures com-bined with contractual increases for inflation, etc. However ... even though D-MACS is paying *more* per patient, our net number of patients is going *down* at a faster rate in this testing market. At this rate, if the trendline here is able to continue, D-MACS will actually exceed cost saving projections by, I'm just guessing here, I'd say by third quarter of this fiscal year. It's working sir. It's definitely working."

Earl grabbed the financial report and flipped back and forth between page seventeen and page twenty-four a few times before allowing a smile to slowly appear on his face.

"I have to present these numbers to members of HHS in a few days on Capitol Hill. Samantha, I expect you to be there to show them what you just showed us. Well done. Is there anything else in these reports of interest to HHS? I mean, they really are a skeptical bunch of bureaucrats. Any morsels that can be tossed their way would keep them off my back for a while."

Samantha flushed, the color rising up her neck and across her cheeks and brow. Fortunately, the cold, icy stares from her colleagues didn't seem to faze her too much. The lady had pluck. "Well, sir, at the risk of sounding presumptuous, I outlined my thoughts in this briefing I brought. The first two pages outline the, um, positive takeaways I think you are wanting."

Earl tapped the side of his nose. The time she spent as a congressional intern also had to have taught her that if the reports didn't have a bulleted outline on page one, no one of any ranking was going to read a word contained in the rest of the report. He'd lucked out with hiring her. Most people thought those in power spent hours poring over research, documents, testimonials, spreadsheets, and anything else to help shape their opinions and views on how to best make informed decisions. Nah. Not at all.

"OK," he said. "So what am I supposed to do with this? What do you recommend?"

Samantha's smile grew wide, reminding him of a pleased cat. He felt a twinge. Power was not necessarily wielded by those with a title. It was in the hands of those who could pull the strings of others without people knowing they were being pulled in one direction or another.

YOU DON'T HAVE TO GO HOME, BUT YOU CAN'T STAY HERE

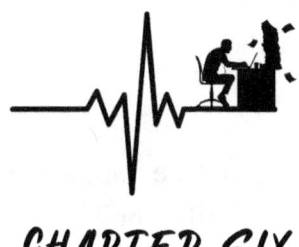

CHAPTER SIX

Evan hadn't shown Peg the Status Quotient algorithm yet. Hell, he hadn't quite figured it out himself, so why bother until he'd fully grasped it. Not that he didn't know *how* to apply the new facet to the calculations—read a table and put in a coefficient. Not hard. What he hadn't figured out was why in the world D-MACS would be shaking up a good thing. Once Evan could grasp a morsel of the "why," he was an ace at putting his full weight behind it.

A staunch company man, Evan aimed to be a dependable resource for any changes in procedure or protocol. Added weight to co-morbidities. Sure thing. Alterations to the prioritization matrix? Bring it on. Even the infamous (many say almost disastrous) modification of the carcinoma scale (known among inner circles as "Cancer-Gate") was easy for Evan. Give him just a crumb, and he'd sell the whole damn cake. But this one? A crumb would have been nice. There wasn't even a whiff for Evan to latch on to. He flipped through his notes from the in-service he had attended and was once again reminded that it was geared toward the "how" while leaving out the crucial backstory that Evan so craved. Having only met the director once (and being underwhelmed and mortified at the same time), he decided to take a chance on going to the source.

Dr. Thompkins's office was located in a large, nondescript governmental office building only a block away from Evan's medium sized, nondescript governmental office building. Rather than take a chance on a phone call ("I'm sorry, Dr. Thompkins is in a meeting right now, can I take a message?") Evan surprised even himself when he left his cubicle.

"Where do you think you are goin', dummy?"

"I ... um ... I'm going to grab some lunch—that new taco truck opened up a few weeks ago and, whew, the line has been crazy. Thought I'd beat the rush."

"Ooooh, yeah. Sounds amazing, my man! Grab me a few of them tacos as well, will ya? I'll pay you back!" Murr had an untarnished record of never paying Evan back for anything.

"Well ... sure, I'll grab you some. Sure thing."

Evan hustled his way through the office, down the elevator, past the security guard, and out onto the street. Once outside, he walked toward Dr. Thompkins's office, immediately second-guessing his attempt at a bold decision. To quiet his indecision, he practiced his opening as he walked.

"Hey, Dr. Thompkins. You probably don't remember me, but I work at D-MACS too."

"I'm Evan—I was at your update the other day. I got a few questions for ya."

"I need some answers, and I need them pronto."

"How you doin'?"

As Evan's attempts at casual banter cliff-dived into an abyss, he stopped in the middle of the sidewalk and debated turning around. "What am I doing? This won't work. This ain't you, Evan. You're not ... (sniff sniff) ... cut out ... (big whiff, now) ... for conflict—hey, is that grilled onions, garlic, and chili powder?"

Evan looked up and realized he was twenty feet from Macho's Tacos food truck. "Well, I can't turn around and face Murr empty handed. And they don't open for another twenty minutes. Shoot. I can do this."

He hurried past the culinary cart and found himself inside the entrance to the office building. Searching the directory, he found Dr. Thompkins's office (Suite 1804), flashed his D-MACS badge to the security guard, and made it to the elevator before he talked himself out of it.

Evan rode the elevator to the eighteenth floor and was decidedly underwhelmed by what he saw when the elevator doors opened. Beigeness and standard issue cheap office art adorned the walls left and right. The reception desk was vacant with no signs of anyone manning it at all (no computer, no phones, no anything). He followed the office numbers down the hallway to the left and hesitated for only a moment before knocking on the door with "1804" stenciled across the frosted glass.

"Come in, it's open!" an older gentleman shouted from behind the door.

Upon entering, a wave of claustrophobia hit him. Piles of folders, books, and papers lay on every square inch of the office. On top of the piles were more piles, many defying all laws of physics by not toppling to the floor. The office was dimly lit with multiple burnt-out fluorescent light bulbs occupying the majority of the ceiling light fixtures. Evan was suddenly put at ease by the woodsy vanilla smell of Three Nuns pipe tobacco hanging in the air. The distinct smell transported Evan back in time to his grandfather's house and the hours spent there. Evan followed the smoke trail to the good doctor.

"Dr. Thompkins?"

"Yes, yes ... I'm back here!"

Evan found a path between the papers that led to the back of the office.

"Hi, Dr. Thompkins. I'm Evan Coleman. I work here at D-MACS too, as a panelist. I'm sorry to interrupt you, but I was hoping to take a minute or two of your time to ask you about your recent presentation."

Dr. Thompkins motioned for Evan to have a seat.

Evan looked around the office for a chair that wasn't buckling underneath the weight of piles of papers and discarded reports but ultimately gave up. "I'll just stand, sir, if that's OK with you. You see, I'm a panelist with D-MACS, like I said, and I'm pretty good at it. But, well, lately I've been struggling with ..."

"Status Quotient. Right?"

"Yes, sir. It's just, to be perfectly frank about it—I mean it's not that it isn't ... what I mean to say is ..."

"Good grief, son ... just spit it out! It's bullshit, right?

The word you're stumbling over, under, and around? Just say it. 'Bullshit.'"

Evan was disarmed, and yet instantly relieved, by Dr. Thompkins's frankness and apparent shared view of this new criterion being introduced. "Yes, sir. It's bullshit—that's exactly what it is. Thank you, sir. So I guess my question is, why? Why did you present it to us if you hate it too?"

Dr. Thompkins chewed on his pipe, then quizzingly stared at it, and then proceeded to go through the same labor-intensive steps Evan's grandfather always went through. All the tapping and refilling and packing and lighting and puffing ... so much work! Evan never figured out why someone would go to all the trouble. Although, for the first time, while watching Dr. Thompkins go through the process, he wondered if that was the actual point of it. The tediousness of the routine must be therapeutic in some way that eluded him. He waited for the doctor to finish his relighting.

Finally, after sending a mighty plume of smoke into the air, Dr. Thompkins sighed. "Well, young man, put it like this. As you go through life, you will seldom ever agree one hundred percent of the time with everything you do or are asked to do. Yet you learn to support it. This happens more often than you think. Happens all the time in relationships. Your wife, girlfriend ... whatever ... asks you to go with her to visit her folks. They're terrible people; you have nothing really in common with them. A ball game you'd rather watch is on—hell, maybe it's your favorite team. In your heart of hearts, you don't agree that going to see her family would be the best use of your time ..."

"But I support it because it's what is best for the relationship?"

"Exactly. Happens at work as well. Your boss says instead of widgets, you'll be making gizmos. Now, you happen to like widgets. They make sense to you. You enjoy making them. You agree with how amazing they are, not only for you, but for the customer base. Gizmos, though? You aren't the biggest fan. You personally would never own one. Yet ..."

"I support it because it's what my employer asks of me?"

Dr. Thompkins puffed on his pipe and approvingly sent smoke towards the ceiling.

"I can certainly see what you're getting at, and I even *agree* with you there, sir. But for me, I need to know the 'why' of something before I can support it ...even if I don't necessarily one hundred percent agree with it, as you said. For your example, maybe gizmos are more popular with different demographic groups, and the company is trying to capture that market. Great. I can get behind that. But how can I support something as deleterious as Status Quotient? I can't get my mind around it."

Dr. Thompkins, instead of responding right away, repeated the process of relighting his pipe. After a few minutes, he turned to Evan with tired eyes and said, "A Malthusianism catastrophe."

Evan blinked. A what now?

"OK. Let's see if I can explain this in a way that helped me 'support' what we are being asked to do here. Are you familiar with Malthusianism?"

Evan shook his head.

"No? OK. I'll put it like this: back in the late 1700s,

Reverend Thomas Malthus hypothesized that technological advances would eventually create a scenario where population growth would outpace things like food production and other resources. Hell, the United Nations predicted that by the end of this century, the population will have grown to a level unsustainable with current resources. Malthus famously said, 'The power of population is so superior to the power of the Earth to produce subsistence for man, that premature death must in some shape or other visit the human race.' Now, I know this theory has been challenged by many as being flawed, but that's what politicians are so good at. And some have taken this theory to inhumane, monstrous levels such as the uptick in eugenics only one hundred years ago. You *do* know it was legal in the United States to sterilize 'undesirable' citizens back in the 1920s, right?"

Evan shook his head, horrified such a thing could have occurred.

"Terrible, terrible time. Ended up sterilizing around sixty to seventy thousand Americans. 'Three generations of imbeciles are enough' said Oliver Wendell Holmes. Terrible time. Hell, even China tried to maintain the one-child policy to decrease population overgrowth. You see how well that worked."

Dr. Thompkins paused, and Evan tried to let everything sink in. His wide-eyed stare and gaping mouth revealed his disbelief and stunned understanding of it all.

"No, Malthus was correct about the dangers of overpopulation, especially without some type of reliable resource management and a coordinated, unified methodology for sustainability. However, I don't subscribe to the notions that have been tried. To paraphrase the saying, 'With great power comes great responsibility,' I like to, instead, say, 'With great *medical* care comes great responsibility.' My mother was kept 'alive,' if you want to call it that, on a ventilator with tubes coming out of every orifice (and a few the medical staff created) to provide her with oxygen, nutrients, antibiotics ... but she wasn't 'alive.' She was a science experiment for soulless doctors."

Tears welled up in his eyes, and he waved them away. Evan shifted uncomfortably, not knowing how to respond to this unexpected display of emotion. He unsuccessfully looked around the office for a tissue.

"Well, kiddo, this is one doctor with plenty of soul to go around, and I don't want to see others go down the same road. Statistically, my mother had no chance, no chance of leading a productive life. While that was almost fifteen years ago, all we've really come up with so far is hospice and palliative care. Well, why even let it get to that level? So, now we have panelists like you, who are truly making a difference in healthcare so we can provide a better chance for those who *can* make it, coupled with a responsible stewardship of our healthcare resources. Unfortunately, the numbers aren't there yet, and I, for one, am not going to let our world starve itself to death. So, yes, as horrible and terrible as Status Quotient seems to me—and obviously you—I think it has its merit in the big picture of how to save this planet." Dr. Thompkins stared at the ceiling and got his pipe back into working order.

"But isn't Status Quotient basically just eugenics with a new label?"

"I don't believe so, kiddo, and here's why: Eugenics, at its core, is the belief that a society should improve the *genetic quality* of the population. Hitler's goal, for example, was to eradicate the Jewish population as he deemed them to be genetically inferior to the Aryan traits. Margaret Sanger and her efforts with birth control have also been tied to her goal of decreasing the black population. Despicable, terrible people. No doubt. Eugenics is flawed and detestable, and I do not support it. Instead, I see Status Quotient as using science, using actuary tables, to better align our goal of getting the right health care to those who will benefit most from limited resources, *regardless* of their genetics. But Evan, at some point, those of us in medicine will have to come to terms with the fact our current system is failing. Our current model is dying the same painful, fruitless death that my own mother went through. I can't allow that to happen. And I bet neither can you."

Evan tried to process this, wishing he had a pipe that needed tending to so he could collect his thoughts. "I don't know, Dr. Thompkins. I mean, I hear you. Loud and clear. But what did you mean by 'the numbers aren't there'? I thought our current process was slowly doing what you are describing. You said, 'getting the right health care to those who it would benefit the most,' right? Well, that's what we are doing. Why drag Status Quotient into the mix?"

The doctor stood and approached Evan, indicating he was ready to walk him to the door. "Because the numbers are not there yet. Another approach was needed, and another approach is what we are doing. We have been hand-picked to be the beta test site for this, and I won't be the one to let this encouraging change die on the vine. I appreciate you coming here, Evan, I really do. I don't often get to talk with those on the front line, and if all panelists are as thoughtful and concerned as you seem to be, I think we are going to do just fine. Thanks for coming in. Thanks."

Dr. Thompkins practically shoved Evan through the door before closing it with a firm click. The suddenness of the director ending the conversation confused Evan and made him consider the true intentions of D-MACS leadership.

Shaking his head, Evan walked to the elevator and pushed the down button. He stood there for a minute, staring at the elevator buttons, wondering if Dr. Thompkins was really delusional enough to believe his own lies.

After grabbing a few tacos, he made his way back to the office, disappointed in his meeting with the director. "There's got to be more to this," Evan told himself as he dropped the Mexican meal on Murr's desk and sat down at his cubicle.

"You didn't get yourself any?"

"Um, I ate mine walking back. So good!" Evan lied through his teeth. Truth is, his stomach was in knots, and he felt more confused than ever. Staring at his computer, he logged back on and hoped his troubled mind would sort itself as he tackled mundane work.

After he removed Evan from his office, Dr. Thompkins stood there, staring at the doorknob, wondering if he'd bought any of it. Because Dr. Thompkins sure as hell did not. He sat down at his desk, relit his pipe, and made the phone call.

She answered on the third ring.

"We got trouble." Dr. Thompkins said into the receiver, puffing a perfect smoke circle above his head. "I think we need to meet."

Hanging up, Dr. Thompkins replayed the conversation with Even in his head and wondered if there was another way. After all, the young idealist panelist seemed so bright and nice. And recruiting new help was getting harder and harder.

He leaned back in his chair and spoke to the ceiling. "That decision is above my paygrade." A ring of smoke drifted up to the rafters. "*Way* above my paygrade."

Peg nervously held the computer mouse and proceeded to log in to D-MACS. This was her first time posting her scores as a full panelist in the system, and she was nervous. "Evan said I was ready," she told herself as the chart appeared before her. "I got this," she repeated to psych herself up. "I got this."

"Let's see. OK. Here we go. Mr. Eduardo Hernandez, #514629799, a fifty-eight-year-old Hispanic male. BMI 34. Ah, yes, too high. History of hypertension, hypercholesterolemia, diabetes ...good grief, it's just about everyone, isn't it? Tonsillectomy as a child, appendectomy at age twenty-three, smoker, moderate drinker, and—oh! What's this? Early onset dementia? Wow, at fifty-eight years old. That's crazy. Presents with new onset shortness of breath to the hospital. Chest X-ray, um, where do I click for that? What in the world? What's empyema? Hover over the word, Peg. OK. 'Empyema is pus in the cavity around the lungs (yuck!) that can be treated with antibiotics and/or surgical drainage'. Hmmm. So, he works as a construction worker and cares for his three children, wife, and grandmother who lives with him. Has he—yes, he's filed his taxes consistently and rents an apartment on the west side of the city. OK, I think he's a solid twenty-seven. Yes, twenty-seven. Let's see, save, post, submit. Done."

Peg stared at the computer screen and waited for her results. Some of her co-workers said they didn't like the consolidated feedback response provided by D-MACS, but Peg liked to check if she was comparable in her scoring with her peers.

"You don't want to be the highest or the lowest scorer," Evan had told her. "Somewhere right in the middle is the sweet spot."

After a few minutes, the feedback response panel posted Peg's score as a solid 52 percent, near the top of the bell curve. "Somewhere right in the middle is the sweet spot," Peg repeated as she patted her right shoulder with her left hand. "Good job, Peg."

She peered around the cubicles with a heightened sense of confidence. None of her fellow panelists seemed to notice her demonstrative self-congratulatory exercise, so she sat there, quietly beaming. First time out the chute and was already feeling good about her progress. Perhaps D-MACS was just the change she needed. Having scored Mr. Hernandez as a twenty-seven, she felt confident he would receive the appropriate healthcare for his condition. Could it be? Could she actually be making a difference in the world? Before clicking on her next chart, she basked for a moment in the afterglow of her job well done.

Shattering her reverie, however, Murray rolled his chair over to Peg's cubicle and grinned at Peg while noisily sucking Cheetos cheese dust off of each finger. "How's it going, Peg?" Murray asked with an orange-dusted smile. "Need any help?"

"Oh, hi Murray. No, no, it's going pretty good. Thanks anyway."

"Well, you know (Murr paused to examine his fingers closely to ensure he had successfully suckled each finger to remove any trace of cheese dust—the ring finger ended up requiring one more round of cleaning), I'm here for ya. Yeah, I'm kind of a big deal around here. Did I tell you I'm usually the one who onboards newbies? I let Evan have a shot at it this time. Yeah, after ten years, I've seen a thing or two." Murr paused to allow Peg time to respond—she didn't—and offered her a Cheeto, which she declined. Well, if you have any questions, let me know. I'm just a cubicle awaaaaaaaay!" Murray said as he scooted his chair back to his cubicle.

Peg stared at the orange trail of dust remaining on the floor from his roll-back to his station. "Ugh."

Keisha, Joanna, Tina, and Charlene leaned out of their respective cubicles to see what was going on. Each had previously occupied that particular cubicle nearest to Murray, and each had gotten permission to move to a more remote location as soon as another cubicle became open. Then they looked at each other with a "been there, done that" expression, shook their heads in sympathy (for Peg) and disgust (for Murray), and slowly leaned back into their cubicles and got back to work.

Peg sighed. At least there was hope one day she too could move cubicles. Apparently, that was more likely than the creep being fired.

Evan nervously held the computer mouse and proceeded to log in to D-MACS. This was his first time posting scores using Status Quotient in the system and he was understandably nervous. "I can do this," he told himself as the chart appeared before him. "I can do this," he repeated to himself to psych himself up. "I got this."

"OK. Mr. Eduardo Hernandez, #514629799, a fifty-eight-year-old Hispanic male. BMI 34, hypertension, etc., etc. Smoker, drinker, presents with shortness of breath, let's see, OK, and empyema. Early onset dementia. So, that makes him, what, about a twenty-seven, twenty-eight? So what about his social determinants? Well, he works in construction, and cares for a wife, three kids, and a grandmother. Apartment, files taxes. OK, this works out good for him, I think. Yeah, his score stays steady (whew!), so yeah. I think he's a solid twenty-eight. Yes, twenty-eight. Let's see, save, post, submit. Done."

Evan was relieved that Status Quotient didn't impact this patient's score. Could it be that using the new variable would not really impact the results as much as he had feared? "Typical Evan," he mumbled. "Always overblowing everything." Filled with relief, he sat there, beaming at his computer monitor. Before clicking on his next chart, he took a moment to silently bask in the afterglow of his anxiety evaporating. His reverie, however, was shattered when Murray leaned his head into Evan's cubicle.

"What about the new girl? Huh? Pretty cute, don't you think?"

"Let this one be, Murr, OK?"

"OOOOOOOOH! You've got a thing for the new girl, is that it?" Murray spun his chair halfway around and pantomimed a serious kiss fest, complete with shoulder caresses and audible lip smacking. "Oh, Peg! You're an animal, Peg! Oh, Peg!"

"Shut up, Murray!" Evan hissed. "There's nothing going on between us!"

Murray suspended his make-believe make-out session somewhere between second and third base and turned back around to Evan. "What did you say?" He flashed an impish grin. "Interesting!"

"Come on, Murr. Cut it out. She's a nice girl. She's sweet. She's going to be an excellent panelist. Don't run this one off, OK?"

"Fine! Good grief, man. Whatever! I'll try to turn down the charm to a solid eight, OK? Jeez! What's up with you, anyway?"

Ensuring no one from management was around, Evan whispered to Murray, "You aren't freaking out about using Status Quotient? It's got me seriously worried."

"Oh, that. Whatever, man. It's just one more dropdown box to click on. What's the big deal? What did you end up giving ol' 'pus in the lungs,' anyway? The new metric didn't change his score at all. You always worry. Remember when we had to add in body weight to the calculation? And you freaked out? What was it you said? 'We're gonna kill them all!' Remember? You're such a dummy!"

Evan stared at the artificial cheese dust creating a John Water-esque mustache on Murray's upper lip and was brought back to reality. What did Harry always say? "Never argue with fools—those around you might not be able to tell the difference."

"You're right, Murr. I was kidding. It's all good." Evan said, attempting to de-escalate Murray's verbal onslaught.

"Damn right, I'm right!" Murray beamed, taking the victory as a win, regardless of his lame so-called argument. "And don't you forget it, man!"

Beaming, Murray rolled backward toward his cubicle. "Not a bad day, my man! I got something spicy cooking with Peg. And I got you to finally admit I'm right—which you should acknowledge more often, by the way." He licked his lips just before backing around the partition and obviously landed on the Cheetos dust mustache. "Ooh, and now I've found leftovers!" He made a show of swiping his tongue around as he disappeared from view.

LIFE, LIBERTY, AND THE PURSUIT OF HAPPINESS

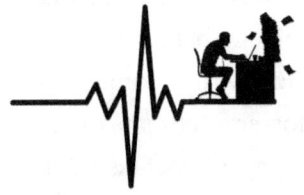

CHAPTER SEVEN

Tabitha McClellan had learned to accept the hand life had dealt her. As a third-generation welfare recipient, she knew the odds were not exactly in her favor. Growing up and living in public housing with her four siblings, she quickly assimilated into the role modeled to her by her mother and grandmother. Tabitha eventually qualified for and received subsidized housing for herself and her two children in the same public housing complex as her mother. Pooling their limited resources and WIC vouchers, Tabitha and her mother felt content in their current setup. Was it perfect? Not exactly. But, as Tabitha often told herself, it could be worse. It would be nice, for example, if her mother would stop encouraging her to get pregnant again in order to increase her government check. Good grief, who in their right mind would possibly want another whining kid? No, she had the ideal set up. Her children shared a room in their two-bedroom apartment and, with her mom only minutes away, she had, essentially, a built-in babysitter for going out when the desire struck her. With her current situation, she had life figured out—life was good.

Tabitha took offense to those who berated her for not having a paid job. Those who cast stones should just try to navigate the parameters that the government tried to implement sometimes. Every time some congressman got a wild hair and tried to foster a "climate of responsibility" among those receiving taxpayer benefits, Tabitha had to figure out new ways to beat the system. Last year it was the healthy-eating initiative. Tabitha laughed out loud at *that* attempt by "the man". Who in the world would want to eat that crap?

A food truck had (briefly) come to Tabitha's complex every two weeks, trying to unload vegetables and who-in-the-world knows what else. Leeks? What were those? Butternut squash? Kale? Don't make me gag! The whole complex eventually banded together and made the food-truck driver steer clear of the housing project. A few well-aimed bags filled with soiled diapers thrown through the driver's side window sent a message loud and clear to the "Veggie-Ville Welcomes YOU" van organizers to "STAY AWAY!"

Yes, Tabitha felt content. Sitting on the front stoop, feeling relaxed after getting both her second and fifth graders on the school bus, she noticed the wildflowers growing in the common area, the result of a group of volunteers who had come through in the summer to participate in a beautification project.

Guilt-ridden volunteers always showed up in the housing projects. "Why do rich people have so much guilt?" Tabitha wondered. It reaffirmed her belief that the saying,

"More money, more problems" was so true that it must be scriptural, right? Looking at the wildflowers, Tabitha knew life really couldn't get much better. Her tranquil moment of transcendental meditation was interrupted by the ringing of her iPhone.

"Yeah, mama, what's wrong now?" Tabitha's mother could be counted on to have something wrong going on at any given point of any day.

"Oh honey, you gotta come quick. I don't think I'm gonna make it. Oh, Lawdy!"

"Mama, mama, now what's wrong? Is it your foot again?" She had a never-healing wound on her right foot from stepping on a piece of glass several weeks ago outside of Miss Llewellyn's complex. And with her high sugar, things just never seemed to heal right with her.

"Oh honey! Oh Lawdy! Yeah, it's my foot again. I fell asleep last night without soaking it in my Epsom salt, and—Oh Lawdy!—it's a throbbin'! I took off my socks and shoes when I woke up, and I just about couldn't stand it! The drainage had plain soaked through my sock, and when I peeled it off, it was bleeding again."

"Mama, I gotta take you to the ER. That's all there is to it, you hear me?"

"Oh honey, no! I don't wanna go back there. They make you sit there for hours and then they try to tell you all kind of foolishness about 'you gotta control your sugar' and 'you gotta eat right' and 'you gonna lose your foot if you don't' kind of talk. I just can't stand that kind of talk, I just can't. Oh Lawdy!"

Tabitha had heard her mother's lamentations about her

ER visit every single day since she took her there six weeks ago. "I'm coming over, Mama. Don't you move."

"How do you expect me to move, Tabby? D'n't you hear me? My foot! Oh Lawdy, my foot!"

Tabitha hung up the phone, grabbed her things, and walked over to her mother's apartment. Before she could knock on the screen door, the odor emanating from her mother's residence just about knocked her over. The combination of rotting fruit ("Can you believe they were throwing this stuff away?"), urine-soaked briefs ("I got the leaky bladder, honey. It'll happen to you one day, y'hear?") and infected drainage from her mother's wound created an overpowering potpourri that made her gag.

"Mama! I'm here, Mama. Where are you?" Tabitha opened the screen door and let her eyes accustom to the dimly lit front living area. Piles of newspapers, magazines, fruit containers, and discarded microwavable food containers prohibited Tabitha from easily seeing where her mother was perched. The smell, however, gave her away. Sitting on the sofa with her foot propped up on the coffee table, Tabitha's mother was rubbing her ankle, rocking to and fro, and moaning over and over "Oh Lawdy" to no one in particular.

The offensive foot in question had soaked through its gauze wrapping onto the table underneath. The purulent drainage, a sickly greenish-gray color, was the clear, undisputed winner of the most-powerful-stench contest, easily winning over first-runner-up rotting fruit and third-place yellowed Depends (although these two were neck and neck). Tabitha, who had not visited with her mother in a few days, was horrified by the amount of drainage.

"I'm calling the ambulance, Mama. Just look at your foot!"

The 9-1-1 dispatcher had a difficult time hearing Tabitha's plea for paramedics over the loud barrage of "Oh Lawdy's" in the background. Finally, after confirming the address, she reassured Tabitha that help was on the way.

Tabitha told her mother she was going to stay on the front stoop in order to direct the paramedics when they arrived. In all actuality, Tabitha was desperate to find a source of fresh air away from her mother's odious appendage. Standing outside, Tabitha felt conflicted about her mother's injury.

On the one hand, Tabitha knew the glass shard her mother had stepped on was from the broken bottle Tabitha herself had thrown (and missed) at her youngest's child's father. Once every three months he would stop in to see his offspring, and once every three months, he and Tabitha would get into a shouting match loud enough to bring out most of the curious residents in her complex. Having derided Tabitha's parenting ("for the last time!"), she had thrown (and missed) the mostly empty bottle of libations in his general direction.

On the other hand, her mother would receive an additional $400 per month should she become disabled due to her foot. She never walked around too much anyways, right? So, in a way, it was gonna help her out.

As Tabitha made her internal closing arguments as to whether or not her mother would be better off with a below-the-knee amputation, the ambulance arrived at the housing complex. She waved the driver down, and it pulled as close as possible to the front stoop, where the two EMTs followed Tabitha into the small apartment.

Terrell never liked calls to public housing. As a child, he visited his now-deceased grandmother in a similar set up. He felt a combination of sorrow for her situation and her acceptance to that fate. Any questions to his parents about it were immediately shut down, so he never got the full story as to her situation. However, he did attribute his work ethic and commitment to self-reliance and bettering himself to this memory. So, in a way, he had to give credit to his exposure as a child in creating his desire to prune this branch of the family tree.

As he and Carlos walked into the apartment with their tackle box, he was immediately knocked over by the smell. Both maintained their professionalism, however, and did a quick assessment, asked a few questions ... then raced each other to the screen door to escape the stench of the malodorous metatarsal.

"Dispatch, this is Shaver, truck 197. We got a sixty-eight-year-old female with a gangrenous right foot. Is a Type II diabetic and has hypertension. No other significant medical history. Right foot wound with copious amounts of purulent drainage. Over"

Standing outside the apartment, Terrell goaded Carlos into making another bet. "Double or nothing. Straight to Regional. I can feel it." After shaking on it, they awaited the call from Central Dispatch. It didn't take long. Once they received direction from the dispatcher, the two retrieved the stretcher from the back of the ambulance and braved the pungent domicile once more. Obtaining a plastic trash bag, they did their best to carefully wrap the foot so as to not elicit rowdier, more raucous shouts of "Oh Lawdy!" from the patient.

"This will keep your mother's foot warmer on the drive to the hospital, ma'am," Terrell dishonestly told Tabitha. In all reality, it was to (hopefully) contain the drainage (and, more precisely, the smell) while in the back of the ambulance.

When everything was loaded up, he told Tabitha that they were taking her mother to Regional General Hospital. Tabitha said she didn't have anyone to watch her children after school and provided her phone number for the emergency department to call her for updates. They got into the front of the truck, and after Terrell started the engine, he reached out his hand to collect his winnings.

Carlos shook his head and focused out the passenger window, his disappointment written all over his face.

After pulling out of the driveway, Terrell nimbly navigated through the projects and slowly headed toward the hospital. The small dose of morphine administered to address the "Oh Lawdy's" was doing its job as Ms. McClellan settled in for the ride to the hospital. No need for the lights or siren; there was no rush where this patient was headed.

The computer cursor blinked incessantly on Evan's computer screen. "I knew it. I *knew* it." It was Evan's first time witnessing the Status Quotient capture its first casualty. His hopes were dashed and his fears realized when he scored the gangrenous right foot a solid seventy-five. A week ago, she would have been an easy forty-two and on her way to getting the help she needed. But with no job, no prospects, and on the government dole, she was now considered too high-risk for D-MACS. For fifteen solid minutes, Evan calculated and re-calculated ... and re-calculated again with the same score. Evan studied the panelists who were up and walking around. No one showed any signs of stress or anxiety, nor were any complaints verbalized from behind the cubicle partitions. Staring at the cursor, he finally submitted his score and sulked back into his office chair.

"How could it have come to this?" Evan paused and focused on the ceiling tiles and fluorescent lighting above his head. His anxiety made his face flush and his heart race while his breathing shallowed. Unable to catch his breath, he stood and walked to the breakroom to collect his thoughts and calm down.

He grabbed a water bottle from the refrigerator and took a long swig. "C'mon, Evan. You got this. Deep breaths." He sat at a table and closed his eyes, trying to get air to his lungs. A chair scraping the floor near him had him jumping and squeaking out a high-pitched "Oh!" His eyes flew open.

Peg screamed. "Oh, my goodness! I'm so sorry! I thought you heard me come in."

"No, no, you didn't startle me. I just, um, hiccupped." Evan tried to recover. "How are you?"

"Well, to be honest, not too good. Did you submit your review of the lady with the infected foot?"

Evan nodded, feeling a sense of relief someone else had qualms.

"It's just not fair, is it?" Her voice was just above a whisper. "I don't understand it."

Inexplicably, Evan felt an obligation to tow the company line and convince Peg that the scoring made sense in the big picture. Perhaps being the devil's advocate for his own strained conscience would somehow subvert his angst.

He found himself repeating most of the talking points provided to him by Dr. Thompkins. It was almost like having an out-of-body experience, floating above the breakroom, his subconscious head shaking at what he was hearing himself tell Peg. The more he rambled, the more disgusted he became with his regurgitation of Dr. Thompkins' lies.

"... may not necessarily agree but be able to support ..."

"... responsible stewardship of our healthcare resources ..."

"... widgets ... gizmos ..."

Peg listened to Evan, her mouth slowly dropping open. The longer he talked, the more her eyes darted around the room. But, for some reason he couldn't shut up. Eventually, she pressed her lips together and bobbed her head up and down, as if agreeing with his words. Yet, he noted, she avoided meeting his eye.

"... so in all actuality, this is what is best for our healthcare at this time." The words fell, hollow and fake, from his lips. Having spent time with Peg while she was being oriented, he had gotten a good idea of who she was, and he sensed that she wasn't buying what he was selling. Her nodding and tacit agreement seemed foreign and ingenuine. Evan knew he had blown it.

In the ensuing awkward silence, Peg blinked her eyes

slowly and cleared her throat. "Well, Evan, that makes a lot of sense. Thanks for helping me understand it better. I, um, guess I better get back to it. See ya." Peg got up and left the breakroom, making as quick an exit as humanly possible.

The warning bells blared in Evan's head as Peg bolted from the breakroom. "What are you doing, Evan?" he mumbled to himself. "Peg's a good person. Why are you trying to confuse her?"

Evan had a calm sense of decisiveness as he realized who would help him make sense of it all. He left the breakroom, logged off his computer station, and made a beeline to the one man who could create some semblance of order to this new era of chaos in Evan's soul.

Samantha smiled to herself after hanging up the phone. Earl Yarborough's words of praise, though not surprising, were nice to hear. His presentation to the Department of Health and Human Services went, in his words, not hers, "as smooth as silk on a shoeshine." Not exactly knowing what that meant, she contextually took it as a compliment, let him know she was glad to have been of assistance, and then hung up. Having established herself as vitally important to the D-MACS CEO went much faster than even Samantha could have predicted. She had given herself a one-year timeline, and having only been in the office for *four months*, she had outperformed even her own vain attempts at humility.

"Smooth as silk on a shoeshine. Yeah, that's me all right!" Samantha said out loud to herself as she locked up her office and made her way to the parking garage. Once in her car, she adjusted the rearview mirror to apply additional lipstick and then smiled at her reflection. "You deserve this, Sam. You go get 'em."

Samantha pulled her car out of the garage and, to her own surprise, made the (unusual) decision to not head straight home. Instead, she made a turn on 17th street to stop at the bar located only a few blocks from her office. Having driven past Houlihan's Hideaway multiple times, she decided to stop in and have a celebration chardonnay before heading for home.

As Samantha walked into the bar, she knew right away she was in the wrong place. Booths lined both sides of the bar and were occupied by a scattering of barflies and lonely Joes who eyed her with equal suspicion. At the bar, a few single occupants were perched on barstools, staring into their drinks, unmindful of anyone or anything around them. In fact, the only real sign of life in the entire "Hideaway" was an older man (who she correctly assumed was the bartender) engaged in a lively conversation with a thirty-something-year-old guy, wearing an unfortunate short-sleeved shirt and even more unfortunate tie. They appeared to be in a deep discussion, with the younger man apparently trying to convince the older barkeep of his side of the argument.

"I'm not going to debate you this. I'm just not."

"As the walrus famously said, 'the time has come to debate many things ...'" the barkeep, surprisingly enough, misquoted to his young debater.

Samantha stealthily attempted to exit the bar before

being noticed when she was flagged down by the aged mixologist.

"Wait, young lady! C'mon in!" The man waved toward Samantha before she could successfully make her getaway.

"As you can see, it's Ladies' Night here at the Hideaway. Please, please, do come in."

Samantha, in all actuality, could never have guessed that, seeing as how the only female in the place was her. She silently cursed her mother's admonition to always be respectful and not rude, albeit traits that had served her well, though in direct contrast to her inner dialogue.

Smiling politely, Samantha slowly made her way to the bar, heading toward a barstool farthest from the quarreling duo when the barkeep stopped her.

"Young lady, my nephew and I are having a disagreement and, if you would be so kind, we would love for an unbiased opinion." He motioned toward where the unfortunate-shirt guy sat. "Now, what'll it be? I can't expect you to make a ruling on our little squabble here without a beverage."

Samantha smiled, placed her order, and proceeded to sit on the barstool.

While the barkeep sang the opening lines to "Margaritaville," the younger man sheepishly smiled. "I'm sorry about Harry. He never met a stranger and likes to make others feel included. My name is Evan."

"Oh, no worries. He seems nice enough. I'm Samantha," she replied, shaking Evan's outstretched hand. "You two sure seemed to be in quite a discussion. I'm really OK to sit over at the other end if you'd like …" Samantha said, gazing longingly toward the barstools farthest from Evan.

"No, young lady—please, I insist. Here's your Mega Margarita—best one in the city, I guarantee you," Harry interjected, pushing the stemmed fishbowl over to Samantha. "Besides, I need to get your opinion on this quandary my nephew here is having with his job."

Evan glared at Harry with no effect.

Ignoring Evan, Harry pressed on. "So, I didn't get your name, young lady."

"It's Samantha," she replied, staring at the drink Harry had placed before her, which was very clearly not the glass of chardonnay she had ordered.

"Samantha. Nice. OK, so here's the situation. Kiddo here has this job with the government. And he's being asked to … what was it again, Evan? What'd you say? 'Violate your principles'? I told him if he is being told to do something by someone above him and that someone is of higher status *in the government*, then whatever it is he is being asked to do must be for a good reason *that is good for us all*. I mean, WE the people vote them into power and they are doing the will *of the people*. And all that jazz!" Harry sang the last few words, complete with jazz hands, to Samantha's surprise and confusion.

She turned from Harry to Evan, not sure what to say. Reluctantly, she asked him a few questions to get more context to his dilemma. Within a few minutes, however, Samantha realized Evan was a panelist and she had the unexpected opportunity to speak with someone "on the front line." Being able to hear from one of the people implementing her pet project of Status Quotient, without him knowing her role at D-MACS, made her smile. She thanked whoever needed thanking for this serendipitous encounter. Feeling as if destiny had coaxed her into this tawdry tavern, she immediately perked up and felt a sense of engagement. Grabbing the margarita, she took a long, thirsty sip and leaned in.

"Tell me more, Evan. Tell me more."

Dr. Thompkins managed to answer the phone on the third ring, recognizing the number right away.

"I just met with your problem boy, Harold. And I think I straightened him out."

Confused, Dr. Thompkins asked Samantha to clarify what she meant.

"The panelist you called me about a few days ago. Evan Coleman. Remember? Had all the questions about Status Quotient?"

Dr. Thompkins knew who she was talking about. He was only hoping she was talking about someone else. He seemed so bright and nice.

"Oh yeah. And exactly how did you 'straighten him out,' if I can be so bold to ask?"

Samantha described in detail the chance encounter at the bar and how she used the bartender/uncle's pretext of "government has our best interest at heart" banter as well as the good doctor's previous conversation to reinforce what Evan should solidify as the truth.

"He never even knew who I was or my association with D-MACS. I mean, it was really easier than I expected. For all he knew, I was just a random person who had an unbiased, 'outsider's' perspective. It was almost too easy! To hit it home, I think you should keep an eye on our idealistic vigilante. Someone like him could really throw a curveball into our new program. I mean, this is going to save our hides, Harold. And I don't have to tell you how that can pay off for us, BIG time."

The promise of a large grant that D-MACS had dangled in front of Dr. Thompkins a few months ago was growing legs, and he was wondering if the payoff was indeed worth the soul selling.

"I certainly understand the importance of these changes, Ms. McAllister. I just don't like the underhandedness of all this. Why, back in my day at the Medical Center in Cleveland ..."

Samantha endured a full thirty-seconds of Dr. Thompkins' sojourn down memory lane before cutting him off.

"Listen, Harold. I've done my part. You just do yours."

After hanging up, he paced back and forth in his office, chewing on his cold pipe, and considering his next move. As a physician, Dr. Thompkins was not entirely comfortable with the new role he was being asked to embrace. Life was so much simpler when he was simply a practicing physician, using evidenced-based medicine to nimbly navigate a patient's health history and clinical presentation to create a pathway for improved health through pharmaceuticals, lifestyle modifications, and carefully crafted therapies. Oh, how he longed for "the good old days" where he could actually use his training and expertise to help his patients.

As Dr. Thompkins mentally unpacked his bag of medical memories, he was abruptly brought back to attention by a *thud* outside of his office. Since he was alone at this time of day, a shiver of fear crept down his spine. He navigated his way around his piles of papers and mounds of mementos to his office door. Upon opening, he looked around and did not see anyone present.

"Hello? Is anyone there?" he asked to no one.

He glanced down and saw a brown, paper-wrapped package at his feet. No writing was on the bundle to clue him as to its sender or its contents. After picking it up, he closed his office door and weaved his way back to his desk, where he placed the package in front of him. He sat in his chair to consider this unusual occurrence. In all of his years, he had never received a mysterious package. He picked it up again and gently shook it, with no sound from within.

"Well, this is curious," he said to himself. "Curious, indeed."

Dr. Thompkins spent the next five minutes attempting to light his pipe as he stared at this new development. Once his pipe was lit, with several smoke plumes rising to the fluorescent lights above, he was ready to face the mystery head on.

He finally opened it and was a bit disappointed to find that it only contained the day's newspaper. However, a cryptic Post-it note piqued his interest. Written in black magic marker was one word:

Obits

Immediately flipping through the paper, Dr. Thompkins easily found the obituary page. As he had gotten older, he found himself following his aged predecessors in making the reading of this section a daily habit—to seek out names he knew, and (as he told others many, many, many times) "just to make sure my name isn't there!"

He had not seen this edition yet, and he slowly read the names listed to find out why he had been instructed to peruse this particular section.

It was then that he dropped his pipe and perspiration dampened the back of his neck. He recognized the name at once and read the full obituary twice to ensure he wasn't mistaken. He wasn't.

Below the picture of his long-time medical colleague, Dr. Simon Corneal, was the usual obituary dribble:

"... beloved husband, father, grandfather ..."

"... active member of many charitable organizations and medical societies ..."

"... medical pioneer at Medical Center in Cleveland before starting a private practice ..."

The final paragraph was what made Dr. Thompkins sit up and feel the cold chill of fear up and down his spine.

"An avid swimmer, the family was devastated to learn of Dr. Corneal's accidental drowning at the Westside YMCA on Wednesday. The family has asked, in lieu of flowers, to please make donations to the YMCA ..."

Dr. Thompkins dropped the paper onto his desk. He had worked with Simon for many years and respected his work and dedication to the pursuit of long-term health through his diet, supplements, and passion for swimming. He would tell everyone who would listen about the merits of swimming, with its cardiovascular benefits, its low-impact muscle building, and its calorie-burning accolades. He was known to swim daily at the "Y" and volunteered for years as a swim coach to underprivileged youth. No way would Simon drown. Impossible.

Dr. Thompkins had seen his former colleague somewhat recently. Simon had been working as a medical consultant for D-MACS for about two or three years, but he never really stayed in touch with him outside of work. When soliciting input into changes, a large group of physicians was routinely used to give scientific validation and approval. Simon was in this group, and he could be counted on to give tacit approval to most papers and briefings. In fact, his last encounter with Simon was ... wait—was that at the Status Quotient presentation? Yes! That was it.

Simon had been vehemently against this newest change, calling himself to the medical approval board a—what was the term? Oh yeah, a "conscientious medical objector" was what he'd said while espousing his reasons for not being able to support "this affront to all we have signed up for when becoming physicians" or something of the sort. When the discussion became more raucous, he'd stormed out of the meeting, yelling to the remaining members of the board, "You all know how I vote on this! May God have mercy on your souls!" He'd even slammed the door behind him.

At the presentation, while talking with some administrators prior to going on stage, he recalled Simon coming up to him and whispering in his ear, "Be careful—they are watching." It was all starting to come back to the director now. As the fog lifted, he recalled that Simon was uncharacteristically disheveled, messy hair, four- or five-day stubble, wrinkled and slept-in clothes. Shrugging it off at the time, Dr. Thompkins had thought his old friend was just trying to rattle him before public speaking. Was he trying to warn him of something? Who was watching? And why was he receiving this obit delivered to his door?

Dr. Thompkins attempted to re-light his pipe but gave up after realizing his hands were shaking so much. Simon was not one for melodramatics or calling attention to himself. In retrospect, he realized Simon had the look of a hunted man. Sitting down at his desk, he dropped his unlit pipe on the papers in front of him. On a yellow legal pad, he jotted down all of these facts and listed out questions that needed answering. These turn of events were not a coincidence and he now felt that maybe poor dear departed Simon was trying to warn him of something more sinister at play. He wished he had connected with him to discuss his concerns instead of dismissing him like the rest of the members of the medical board. Staring at the pad of paper, he reviewed his list and realized how naive he had been and how he had not considered all the downstream (and upstream) players involved in this newest D-MACS development and apparent threat. Not knowing his next steps, he decided leaving the solitude of his office was the safest idea. After grabbing his coat and pipe, he placed his yellow pad and various journals and papers in his briefcase and made a quick exit, double-checking the locks on his office door. After all, one could never be too careful, right?

MISERY SURE LOVES COMPANY, DON'T IT?

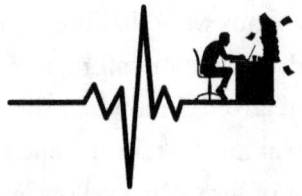

CHAPTER EIGHT

After twelve seasons of *What's Cookin', Good Lookin'?* Chef Pierre Beaumont had grown bored. And lazy. And fat. Really fat. It really wasn't his career plan to become an instantly recognizable celebrity TV chef, but here he was, killing it. Quickly rising through the ranks in cooking schools, and then becoming, seemingly overnight, the owner and Chef de Cuisine of not one, not two, but three 3-star Michelin restaurants, he decided to hang up his toque and host the immensely popular cooking show. Like everything else in his life, success had come remarkably easy for him. It was almost inconceivable to him that people actually watched him season after season make, in his mind, the simplest of dishes. Pancetta with legumes? Easy-peasy. Yorkshire pudding? Yawn. Wagyu beef with white truffle sauce? Whatever. He never really understood why it was so easy for him. But, good grief, people really ate it up. Literally. And having a movie-star quality face didn't hurt his meteoric rise either.

When he was pitched the show by a television producer who was enamored by his take on remoulade, he was ready for a change and thought it might awaken a challenge within him. It didn't. Coming out to the studio audience's thunderous applause, he would shout the catch phrase, "What's Cookin'?" to the crowd, to which they would feverishly shout back, "Good Lookin'!" to Pierre. He became even more wealthy than he had already been, and then came the merchandise. Aprons. Cookware. Cooking utensils. Coffee mugs with his own mug printed under the catchphrase sold like hotcakes.

But without a challenge, he quickly grew bored. His contract, which he never bothered to closely read, was for fifteen seasons of the show. By season five, he was ready to quit and was given the shocking news by his agent that he was only one-third of the way through his contract. Stuck, he let his boredom seep into his appearance, and, unfortunately, his cooking. Like all celebrities, if you didn't stay hungry, you lost your edge.

Pierre missed tapings due to oversleeping, the result of overindulgence in food-delivery services. More than once, Chef Beaumont had had to slam the door in the face of a pimply-faced delivery boy saying, "Hey! Ain't you that celebrity chef? Yeah, yeah! You're that *What's Cookin'* guy, ain't cha? What are you doing ordering Burger Buddy? I mean, you could cook ..." *SLAM!* Right in his face. As a result, the television studio had insisted that Pierre's agent arrange for a handler to wake him up, drag him into an icy shower, and get him to the studio in time for make-up to *try* to bring back that "Good Lookin'" face to some level of recognition. However, no amount of foundation, pancake makeup, or concealer could reverse the damage he had done. Chef Pierre Beaumont had unfortunately lost his allure, as one might say. Most comparisons (which Pierre had grown tired of) were of Marlon Brando "near the end" ... only heavier.

Having ballooned to a weight of 387 pounds, Pierre's girth had grown to gargantuan proportions. His nimble hands, which had previously and effortlessly diced, minced, and chopped, were now all but useless, having turned into two ham hocks with ten plump sausages attached. The television studio was forced to use "hand doubles" for the close-ups of Chef Beaumont preparing dishes. As for the studio audience, they were unaware all ingredients were pre-prepared to accommodate Pierre's inability to safely handle cooking knives anymore. He was a mess and had turned into a Macy's Thanksgiving Parade float caricature of his former glory days. C'est la vie, no?

Devon Robinson was thrilled ... no ... ecstatic ...no, thrilled was the right word, thrilled to land the job of being Chef Beaumont's handler three months ago. To be able to be *right there* with a living legend! Wow! While his mom didn't understand the job duties exactly, she was proud of him to have a steady job, nonetheless.

"Why does a grown man need someone to help him put on his tighty-whities? I don't get it."

"MOM! I don't just assist him in his wardrobe for the day! Jeez!"

"I don't get it, Devon. They are paying you all that money to do what exactly?"

"I am Chef Pierre Beaumont's personal assistant, OK? He is a busy man, top of the food chain (so to speak) in the culinary world. And I am there to assist him with arranging transportation, shopping, light cleaning, answering correspondence, y'know … the day-to-day things in life that he can't be bothered with. Jeez!"

"And helping him put on his tighty-whities, right?"

"Jeez!"

After three months of helping Chef Beaumont struggle in and out of his underwear, he regretted pleading with his mother to stop denigrating his job.

"Why in the hell am I getting paid to help a grown man put on his underwear?"

The money was good.

Hey, the money was reeeeaaaal good. After a few weeks, Devon had created a system to save his sanity and get Chef Beaumont to the church on time (well, the television studio). Using the good chef's American Express card, he had coordinated a team that Devon would stack up against any high functioning military operation. Cleaners, laundry services, new clothes to be delivered every three days (consisting of XXXL briefs, T-Shirts, and sleepwear), bed pads, and, to Chef Beaumont's delight, a constant delivery of snacks, fruits, crudités, chocolates, and pastries (from Auberge Patisserie on 7th, no less). The timing and precision Devon had devised was, in his opinion, sheer poetry. It was a bit of a pain to have each delivery person and cleaner sign an NDA, but it turned out no one really cared about Chef Beaumont in this circle of workers anyway. It was a fine thing and a work of art. All Devon had to do was show up and orchestrate the music, keeping each instrument in time and in check.

When Devon showed up at seven o'clock on Thursday morning to begin the day, he felt a sense of pride and accomplishment for having landed this job. He no longer viewed the job as an exercise in futility as he had just about farmed out all the unsanitary, unseemly aspects of the role to others.

Except for one—a lone holdout task that Chef Beaumont refused (threw a tantrum, more like it) to have anyone else participate in. He seemed to have developed a reliance on Devon that grew into trust and, after three months, more of a comfort and reliable routine. Having lost control of his bodily functions several months ago, Chef Beaumont required immediate and thorough cleaning upon awakening, with his night clothes and underwear being double bagged into industrial strength trash bags and having his bed linens quickly removed and placed in a hamper for laundering.

This process was mortifying for Devon at first, but, like most things in life, one can learn to do just about anything with the proper preparation and mental acumen. Entering Chef Beaumont's bedroom, Devon no longer reeled from the odor of excrement that filled the chambers. Having seen one of his grandmother's favorite medical shows, he got the idea from a pathologist performing autopsies to use oil of wintergreen under his nostrils to block the smell. If it was good enough for Quincy, then it should be good enough for Devon, right? With a couple of crucial drops under each nostril, Devon was able to safely put up with whatever the good chef could put out and not suffer from the dry heaves.

Standing outside of Chef Beaumont's bedroom, Devon prepared himself, opened the door … and promptly threw up his breakfast. Due to the darkness of the bedroom, Devon wasn't quite sure what he was seeing, but he sure knew what he was smelling. The two drops of oil of wintergreen didn't even begin to combat the odor assailing his senses. Adjusting his eyes to the darkened room, he tentatively reached for the master switch to shed some light on the situation. As he tried to take it all in and make sense of it all, he realized that this time Chef Pierre Beaumont was beyond Devon's control. Dialing 9-1-1, he decided to bring in the professionals.

"**Gather 'round, everyone!** C'mon, c'mon. This is big time. We got ourselves a Code Orange alert here … yeah, you heard me. Code Orange. C'mon. Murray! Get over here!"

Having worked for D-MACS for the past thirteen years, Theodore Butler had seen just about everything. Rising through the ranks as a panelist, he became the shift supervisor, the highest-ranking administrator on the floor, three and a half years ago. Many days—more like *most* days—Theo's responsibilities were relegated to ensuring that the panelists submitted their chart reviews in a timely manner and reviewing any wayward tabulations with the specific panelist outlier. Over the last few years, Theo had helped mold a well-working team that, for the most part, tabbed very similar reviews. Oh, he had to reign in Murray from time to time, but that was more of a personality issue than a job function concern. Theo was not very liked by most of the panelists but, hey, this wasn't no popularity contest. By now, most of the panelists could finish his mantras as if they were etched in stone.

"Get your reviews done on time!"—"*If we don't, it's a crime!*"

"When in doubt?"—"*Give Theo a shout!*"

"If a patient is in need?"—"*D-MACS is there indeed!*"

(OK. For the record. That one was Theo's least favorite, but he came up with it in case senior leadership were to ever make an appearance on the floor and he could demonstrate his loyalty to the organization. This one elicited the most eye rolls from his direct reports, but, again, this wasn't no popularity contest!).

As each of the panelists came together for the huddle, Theo paced back and forth, causing a few of the panelists to whisper to each other their theory on whom the Code Orange was being called for.

"I bet it's what's-his-name, the rapper who just moved to town. You know they all do the drugs."

"Uh-huh. Or, hey, who's the lady with all those interior design shows? I heard she does the drugs too."

"You guys are nutso. My money is on the governor. All red faced and full of stress. He's a cardiac arrest just waiting to go off!"

Theo tried his best to reign in the agitators. "OK, OK. I think everyone is here. No, no, no. Stop the rumors. I hear you all mumbling under your breaths. We have a Code Orange here, folks. A Code Orange."

Several of the newer panelists looked quizzically at each other.

"I realize many of you have never had a Code Orange

so let me give you the scoop. As you know, we divide up the patient cases that come in among you, and each of you do a great, and I do mean great, job of tabbing your reviews in a timely manner. I don't have to tell you, senior leadership is just really, really pleased with the new numbers you all are submitting. Being the beta testing site for Status Quotient wasn't the most popular with many of you, but, hey, that's OK. I, myself, am proud we were selected to try it out. Us! That's saying something, you know? But, I get it. Change is hard. Especially for some of you more than others."

Theo stared at Evan as he spoke, and he noticed a flush creep across his face as his eyes darted over to Peg. He momentarily wondered if there was something going on between the two panelists, but simply dismissed it as his own overactive imagination.

"No, this Code Orange is in reference to #61328346, which is about to come into some of your inboxes. I'm not sure which of you will get this case assigned to you by the system, so I wanted you all to be aware. This is a special case that will require my approval before submitting due to its, um, delicate nature. If you are assigned this Code Orange, I want you to review the case and then meet me in the conference room in, what, six minutes? The rest of you, get back to your other reviews and stop the rumor mill. You all will find out soon enough. C'mon, people! Move it!"

Everyone moved back to their cubicles and each panelist eagerly waited to see who would be assigned the review.

Theo had gotten the call from Central Dispatch who had been alerted to the call from Chef Pierre Beaumont's residence just a few moments prior. Like most uber-celebrities, each of their residences were kept on a separate server for when an emergency 9-1-1 call came in. In order to head off paparazzi or other unscrupulous news hounds, calls on this select list were treated differently than others and went straight to a designated dispatcher who was trained to handle the situation delicately. As such, a heads-up call was placed to D-MACS in order to ensure expedited reviewing, and an immediate direction was expected to be provided pronto. While the randomly selected panelists reviewed the chart, Theo went to the conference room to pull up the needed computer monitors and screens, awaiting their arrival.

It did not take long for the four panelists to file into the room with Theo. Evan arrived first, followed by Tina, Joanna, and then finally Murray. Murray was the first to break the tension.

"Ha-ha! I told you all, didn't I? Didn't I tell you that chef dude was gonna drop any day now? Ha-ha!"

"Ok, Murray, keep it down. Let's start with you, Evan, what are your thoughts on this?"

Evan took control of the computer mouse and highlighted various aspects of the good chef's patient chart. "Well, based on his BMI, history of diabetes, hypertension, etc., presenting with colon perforation, I would score him a solid sixty-three. But ..."

The other panelists nodded as Evan minimized one screen and toggled to the Status Quotient section.

"But ... and I haven't encountered this yet, but based on the Status Quotient due to his notoriety and income, his score is reduced to ... to a thirty-one? Is that right?"

Theo had anticipated questions from the group as most

of the newest tabulations that panelists were experiencing with Status Quotient were taking mild to moderately sick patients and increasing their scoring due to lack of, essentially, a bright future. Homeless, jobless, not really contributing to the "greater good." Although Theo was keenly aware of some of the rumblings among his panelists, they had each fallen into lock step fairly well, even Evan who, at first, showed the most visible signs of pushback or virtue signaling with his peers. Theo, himself, was most concerned about this addition by D-MACS but was relieved to see that relatively few ripples developed within the team. However, he had justifiably dreaded the team's first exposure to using Status Quotient to give the impression of a leg up to someone of wealth or notoriety.

"OK, OK. Yes, that would be the appropriate utilization of Status Quotient for this patient." The four panelists sat back in their chairs and crossed their arms in a uniform display of disapproving solidarity.

"Let's quickly level set here as a reminder of what we all were taught recently by Dr. Thompkins. Yes, this patient is benefitting from this scoring system. But also, think of how many others are benefitting as a result of this score. Those who the chef employs, for example. Those in the television studio. Those in the merchandising business. I don't need to remind you, but many, many people's lives would be negatively impacted should the good chef not make it. So, let's do the right thing here."

Theo reached across the table and, taking the computer mouse from Evan, saved and submitted the score before there could be any more discussion.

Tina and Joanna each raised their hands in unison.

"Yes, Tina?"

"Joanna and I have just one quick question, Mr. Butler."

Theo gave a long pause before responding. "OK. What is it, Tina?"

Tina winked at Joanna and let out a small snicker before asking. "Do you think Status Quotient is gonna save you or hurt you when *your* time comes?"

Theo remained silent as one by one the four panelists got up from their seats and filed out of the conference room. Evan was the last and turned back to Theo before exiting.

"Good for the chef. Bad for the rest of us."

The door closed behind him and Theo sat alone with his thoughts in the conference room. He knew he was required to make a phone call after the first Code Orange. But he wanted a few moments to consider the consequences being unleashed with his guidance. Finally, Theo grabbed the phone and dialed.

She answered on the second ring. "Well, it could have gone better."

"Tell me more, Theo, tell me more."

Samantha felt unsettled. She knew Dr. Thompkins and was satisfied with the conversation they had, as well as the not-so-subtle message that the untimely death of one of his colleagues surely must have had on him. As he had not reached out to her lately, she considered it a sign that he understood his place in the organization as well as his purpose for achieving this greater good. Samantha also felt satisfied with her chance meeting with Evan Coleman at the local bar. Her conversation with him gave her the confidence that he was going to be a team player and was, at heart, a true company man who might just be key to ensuring that this beta testing site for Status Quotient came through in the clutch. It wasn't Dr. Thompkins. It wasn't Evan. Then what was it, Sam?

It was the damn phone call from Theodore Butler. Except she had anticipated the call, so what was it? Was it the fact that a person of wealth and status benefitted from the new variable in calculating medical regimen recommendations? Nah. Hell, she had envisioned it and helped create the nuances of it with the assistance of a few code writers. And D-MACS would soon be reaping the reward of her hard work. You know what it was? It was the last thing Theo said before hanging up. What was it? "Well, they went along with it ... this time." What did *that* mean? "This time"? Why would the panelists have reservations? It was the most meticulously well-scripted, thought-out coup de grâce that could have ever been added to the current formulary. "This time"? Give me a break. She had never met this Theodore Butler, but obviously he wasn't conveying the buy-in and sense of confidence needed at this crucial testing and implementation time.

Samantha paced back and forth in her home office to get her creative juices flowing. Talking out loud to herself, she was able to brainstorm her next steps. This combination of activity with "talking it out" had never let her down before.

"Dr. Thompkins is my ace in the hole for bringing medical credo to all these changes. Check. He's on board, and I got him scared. This Evan guy, he is towing the line and will do what is told of him. Check. Theodore Butler, however, is the grunt that is supposed to bring administrative clout to the panelists. He tripped up on this one and couldn't score the lay-up, despite having the information and the sense of urgency. *He*'s the problem child here. I think a visit from the good doctor will shore up his reservations and help him to understand what is at stake here."

Samantha stopped pacing and felt good about her decision. She picked up the phone, told Dr. Thompkins what to do, and then promptly opened a bottle of Cabernet she had in her wine refrigerator. Holding her glass up, she admired the Marangoni effect of the wine legs resulting from her gentle swirling of the cab. She guessed the alcohol content of this bottle to be 14.5 percent based on her assessment of the larmes de vin. Checking the bottle, she confirmed her guess, then raised her glass in a toast to the good doctor. "Here's to you, doc. Here's to you. Now, seal the deal."

Dr. Thompkins felt unsettled. "What am I doing?" he asked as he peered out his office window, having just hung up the phone with Samantha. "What am I doing?"

He had always found solace in his research and in trusting the science. In all of his years in medical practice, he had never felt these new feelings of tension and anxiety. Over the decades, he had provided some of the best care known to Western medicine, never wavering in his firm belief of medical ethics and of what was just. He had always been able to justify in his mind any decision made for his patients. What about his role with D-MACS was creating such upheaval in his soul?

When he was asked to join D-MACS, first as a medical advisor, and then as the medical director, he was told that he would be the voice of reason in a world of ever-changing priorities and principles. When in doubt, Dr. Thompkins was always able to use *science* to sustain him and guide his path. He had served on various boards and councils, elevating his status among his peers as one who kept the torch of patient's rights burning bright. In fact, it was Dr. Thompkins who served on the board several decades ago to help determine what principles should be used when developing the framework for how to best care for patients. This created the first foray into what is now widely utilized in the realm of Medical Ethics. These principles ensured that patients were treated with dignity, kept from harm, and had equal access to resources.

"Ensure that resources are distributed equally among all patients." Dr. Thompkins abruptly sat in his chair and considered how far he had strayed from this tenet of medical ethics that he had once held so true. "What am I doing?" he asked again.

He grabbed his pipe and began the process of adding tobacco and getting it lit while he sat in silence. This combination of relighting his pipe with sitting in silence had never let him down before.

As the first series of smoke rings circled his head, he thought about how far he had come. He wondered if he could stay true to his medical training to care for patients while still influencing the delivery of care in the current climate of medical uncertainty. The pit in his stomach answered his question and substantiated his self-doubt.

Peg had never been much of a cook. Now don't get her wrong, she could nuke a mean SimpleStuff frozen dinner. Not too hot, not too cold. Just right. And she stayed tried and true to her "secret" for keeping microwave meals moist while being heated. A wet paper towel. A say what? Yes, a slightly damp paper towel to essentially steam the food in tandem with the magic of the microwaves. Or whatever it was that provided the source of heat. All she knew is that her 150-calorie Veggie-sagna was hot, not dried out, and as delicious as a 150-calorie Veggie-sagna can get. Staring at the half-eaten meal, she couldn't bring herself to finish it. Whenever Peg was anxious, stressed, or worried about something, her "tell" was a lack of appetite. Her attempts to pump herself up fell flat.

"Today I seized the day. Today was mine to conquer. Today was ..." What was today, Peg? Huh? Today was tough. It was terrible to see Evan look so broken. Since starting at D-MACS, Peg enjoyed seeing Evan in the office, occasionally getting a cup of coffee in the breakroom at the same time as him and discussing nothing of any real significance. Except it *was* of real significance to Peg to have these exchanges. Fewer and fewer good ones were out there, and Peg was confident he was one of them. He was so patient with her during her training, and he seemed to really care about his role in D-MACS. But today was bad. She knew it had to have been bad, watching him walk out of the conference room, saying something to Theo and then closing the door firmly behind him. As he walked back to his cubicle, she considered the thousand different thoughts she'd seen flit across his worried face.

Peg decided to make Evan homemade cookies to ... well, maybe they'd lift his spirits some. Peg searched through her refrigerator for the "Break N' Bake" cookies she had bought a week or two (or three) ago. As she searched for the half-eaten package (Peg was known to "break n' eat" the raw dough on occasion), she preheated the oven. Next came the cleanest dirty cookie sheet she could find in her kitchen, onto which she placed the remaining break-apart cookie-dough blobs.

Setting her timer, she mused on the events of late at the office. In her short few weeks there, Peg had felt a real sense of purpose, something she had never really felt in any previous job. This was important stuff they were doing, right? Change the world stuff, yeah? Being a part of a team felt amazing, and she was troubled to see any disruption to this sense of unity and camaraderie that she felt a part of for the first time. Why would anyone want to destroy that?

The timer dinged. After carefully removing the cookies from the oven, Peg placed them on the counter to cool. Staring at them, she felt a sense of accomplishment, and her uneasiness dissipated. "Yes, these will make Evan feel better and let him know that he's in the right place. I just bet they will." Cookies could solve just about anything.

A CHANGE WILL DO YA GOOD

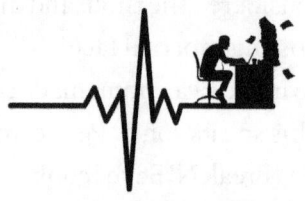

CHAPTER NINE

Evan went through his normal routine to get ready for work. He had used the same brand of shaving cream his father had bought for him at the first sign of peach fuzz ("Hey, honey! Come check out the newest member of ZZ Top before he shaves it all off!"). He even used the same soap he was brought up on ("Aren't you glad you use Dial? Don't you wish everybody did?"). In fact, very little in Evan's daily routine had not been perfected at least twenty years ago. Same shower routine (wash hair, rinse, repeat), same dressing routine ("Of course I put on my right sock, *then* my left sock, *then* my right shoe, *then* my left shoe. You think I'm crazy?"), and the same breakfast routine. Well, in all fairness, this is where sometimes Evan went a little wild. He had Nature's Granola cereal every Monday (of course). But every now and then, Evan felt the pull to be spontaneous and would add some Oat Bran to the same bowl! Like a two-fer! Cray-zee!

But that's about as much wild-abandonment as Evan's heart could stand. He was the first to admit it. He liked the same old, same old. A certain level of comfort could be found in the mundane. Who wanted the chaos that change could bring? Not Evan! And for all these years, Evan knew he could count on his job to be as unchanging, as unwavering, as constant as, well, as Evan's tooth-brushing routine ("You gotta start on the right side, top teeth. You just gotta!"). So why was D-MACS trying to muck everything up now?

Yesterday was awful, and Evan felt a flurry of emotions thinking about it. His sense of fairness was upended. His faith in "the greater good" was turned upside down. His level of respect for Theo ... well, that hadn't really changed too much, had it? Theo was a toady and would only do whatever his superiors expected of him to not rock the boat. In fact, he often said as much: "C'mon, guys! Don't rock the boat! This is what the senior team has decided. Now, c'mon!"

Evan was not one for conflict. No sir. Now, however, Evan felt empowered by his convictions like he had never felt before. Maybe it was the "two-fer" cereal he had this morning talking, but he had a real sense of revolution in his heart and mind as he put on his right shoe, then his left shoe. Yes, Evan had decided. He was going to get in there and ... and—sitting back down on his kitchen barstool, he realized he had no idea what he was going to do about this new sense of disruption and corporate agitation welling up inside him. No, he wasn't sure at all, and his shaking hands belied the bravado with which he had stirred up his mind. "What to do, what to do?" he repeated as he cleaned up his breakfast bowl, ensuring the counter was free of any spilled milk or cereal crumbs. "What to do, what to do?" he chanted, and then, as he grabbed his keys, he realized that, yes, in fact, for the first time in many, many years, he knew just what to do.

Carlos Diago turned to Terrell as they pulled up to the residence where the 9-1-1 call had originated. Before he could say anything, Terrell jumped in.

"I'll bet you fifty bucks this one goes to Regional General. Fifty bucks."

Carlos Diago countered. "Baloney. This is the uptown district. Gotta be some money here, man! No way they gonna send us past Sherman Memorial to go to Rege. No way!"

"Put your money where your mouth is, my man! I'm telling you. This may be uptown *to you*, but it ain't no uptown to D-MACS. Uh-uh. We goin' to Regional General. You watch."

"You don't even know what's wrong with this one. Could be a sprained ankle or sumfin'."

"Well, that's why it's called gamblin', 'Los. Whatcha say? Fifty?"

"You gotta bet, sucker."

Carlos had worked with Terrell Shaver on Ambulance #37 for the past two and a half years and, admittedly, had learned a few things from him in that time. Some of what he learned was clinical, with more real-world techniques for handling broken bones, for example, or how to tell a drug seeker looking for a morphine hit from a true chest painer. Yeah, Terrell had been around the block a time or two and had seen just about everything under the sun. Carlos knew Terrell was probably right about the hospital, but it was good to let someone win every now and then just to keep them in your good graces. Lord knew it was anyone's guess anymore where dispatch would end up having them haul their pick-ups. Terrell had caught on pretty fast with this new routine and it did seem that the better the zip code, the better the chances of going to a closer hospital.

As Carlos and Terrell walked into the entryway of the residence (*An entryway? YES! I knew it! My money is safe!*), they got straight to work on the patient lying on the couch. (*Is that suede? Fifty bucks in the bag!*) After quickly assessing the situation, Carlos started an IV and initiated a bag of Lactated Ringers while Terrell gave the patient a sublingual nitro pill and had him chew an aspirin. While Carlos hooked up the EKG, Terrell called it in.

"Yeah, dispatch. We got a fifty-five-year-old white male, diaphoretic, vitals OK except for a BP of 178/96. Complainin' of chest pain with radiation to left arm and neck. Yeah, we are doing the EKG now. It's just about ... yeah, here it is. Those are some tombstone T-waves if I ever did see it—see that Carlos? Yeah, uploading to you now. It looks like an acute MI to me. Where you wanna us go? What? OK, call me back. We'll start loading him up."

They made quick work of getting the patient on a stretcher, and Terrell's phone rang as they were just reaching the front door.

"Shaver here. Yeah. OK. Got it." Terrell smiled a big smile at Carlos.

He knew what that smile meant. How'd Terrell know? It sure seemed like a pretty nice neighborhood compared to Carlos's dilapidated duplex. Oh well, easy come, easy go. At least Regional General had better fast-food restaurants near it. Plus, maybe he could get Terrell to go double or nothing.

Hitting the lights and siren (as instructed) as they wound through the neighborhood, they made haste until reaching the main road. Once there, they killed the lights (again, as instructed), then took their time en route to Regional General. Little chance this heart attack was going to make it with the extra distance and time needed to get all the way across town to Regional, but, D-MACS knew what they were doing, right?

The big smile on Earl Yarborough's face almost made his cheeks hurt. But he couldn't help it.

"Damn, that Samantha was right."

The latest numbers for the beta testing site that had come in were right on the money. Literally. Admits were down. Dollars spent were down. And Earl felt an almost childish giddiness in thinking about how he was going to be spending his bonus.

Putting the financial report down, Earl picked up the "Yachts and You" catalog and turned straight to the dog-eared page that he had looked at longingly over and over the past few weeks with unabashed enthusiasm. He really didn't have to read the details on its specs as he had memorized them already. But he couldn't help himself by reading them aloud anyway, just for fun.

"The 64 Excalibur Convertible Yacht: Sporting fun combined with sun-kissed prestige for the avid boatsman!"

Earl scanned the details in the pictures contained in

the catalog, envisioning himself at the helm. He had always wanted to be thought of as an "avid boatsman." He could almost taste the salty sea breeze as he imagined himself being the envy of everyone at the boat club.

And, ahem, the bikini-clad little number lounging on the sundeck of the cruiser didn't hurt the allure either. Earl was *pretty sure* she was not included in the hefty price tag ... but he anticipated that someone of equal caliber would be more than willing to join him on the water for some maritime merriment. After all, Gladys hated the water and was more than willing to NOT join him in order to spend more time at the country club with her tennis and her massages.

All because of this Samantha and her spot-on decision to make some changes to D-MACS. Earl was more than pleased to have someone else do the heavy lifting and make him look good for a change. In all of his years at the top of D-MACS, Earl couldn't remember a better time in his career. The board was off his back thanks to the newest promises that the beta testing site was showing. The bean counters were not breathing down his neck to tighten up this or cut back on that. Even the dimwits up on Capitol Hill seemed to be giving him "attaboys" more than ever, thanks to the great financial outlook he took credit for. After all, Earl had put together the right team to make the hard decisions for him. He couldn't be bothered to also develop every initiative or nuance that came his way—that's what he paid others to do, right?

Feeling good for the first time in years about how things were going, he sat back in his upholstered desk chair, smiling to himself. Then, Earl called for his assistant through the intercom on his desk.

"Yes, Mr. Yarborough?"

"Dotty, do me a favor, will ya?"

"Yes, Mr. Yarborough?"

"Send a floral arrangement for me to that Saman-tha McAllister, will ya? Have the card say something like, 'Thanks for all the hard work - I appreciate you' or some-thing. You'll make it sound good, won't you Dotty?"

"Yes, Mr. Yarborough."

"Thanks, Dotty."

"Yes, Mr. Yarborough."

Releasing the intercom button, Earl picked up the Yacht catalog and stared again at details of the 64 Excalibur. Yes, things were going very well for Earl Yarborough. And it didn't look like anything was on the horizon to cause him any heartburn.

Which is why the incessant pain Earl felt across his chest was so damn annoying. Rubbing his chest with his right hand, he opened the top drawer of his oak desk and grabbed a couple of antacid tablets. Quickly chewing on them, Earl decided to start eating healthier. As the indigestion dis-sipated, he patted his enormous expanse of a waistline, acknowledging that he could stand to drop a pound or two. After all, the cutie who would soon be lounging on *The Sea Sweet* sun deck would probably like that as well. And who was Earl to disappoint?

As Carl loaded his Keurig Coffee Maker (*"Donut-Shoppe" flavor—yum!*), he turned to Bill and said, "How are you feeling about all this?" Carl was confident in his role as assistant lead evaluator for D-MACS at Regional General but was woefully inept at reading the tea leaves when it came to the future in his role. Not to say that he wasn't great in his job, he just wasn't wired to see how changes to routine or processes would pan out. He relied heavily on Bill to realign his moral compass to orient him back to true north. As the lead evaluator for D-MACS, Bill was well versed at taking whatever mandates were thrown at them and making lemonade, so to speak.

With Status Quotient continuing into the testing phase, the patients now coming to Regional General were even more polarized in their presentation. The ones who came in by ambulance with lower scores, by and large, were healthier and more likely to have a positive outcome. However, more and more patients were arriving with higher scores and, conversely, did not have such positive outcomes. These required carefully scripted conversations with their families.

"Of course the team is devastated that Mr. Jenkins didn't survive the surgery, ma'am."

"The extent of her illness was extensive and contributed to her passing, Mr. Palmer."

"Everyone at Regional General extends their condolences and wishes you peace during this difficult time, Ms. Roberts. Do you have a funeral home preference? If not, here is a list of excellent ones in the area."

Notoriously nonplussed, Bill took it all in stride and saw each change as just another typical day in healthcare.

"I'm feeling good about everything, Carl. Real good. Why?"

As Carl blew on his cup of coffee, he marveled at Bill's ability to never show stress or disenchantment with his job.

"No reason. Just checking in with you. I mean ... well, I guess I was just asking 'cause it seems like we have less and less to do most days, doncha think? I mean, the patients come in either pretty healthy or, well, since a lot of the sick ones are sicker, they come in ... mostly dead, y'know? Don't you think we could be out of a job soon at this rate?" Carl's propensity for pessimism and worry was annoying to many—he'd been told— but not Bill, who really liked the role of comforter, which Carl appreciated.

Wanting to be helpful, in case their jobs were in jeopardy, he pulled out a few brochures from the local funeral homes and held them up to Bill. "I picked up a few of these the other day. Ted down at Pulaski and Sons said they're hiring. Said they are busier than they've ever been and are looking for help."

Bill's disapproving expression had Carl sheepishly adding, "I mean, we kind of already act like a funeral parlor attendant most days now ..." He trailed off, under the weight of Bill's icy silence, strongly wishing he had not suggested anything. Feeling large and awkward, he shifted his weight from one foot to the next and then back again.

Finally, Bill gave a big, warm smile showing off how straight and polished his teeth were. "I don't think you need to worry about hunting for other jobs, Carl. I have it on good authority that D-MACS is more than pleased with how well we've been navigating these changes. And *you*, Carl, you are doing just amazing with it all. I mean, come on, remember how well you handled the Samson family this morning?"

With a pat on Carl's back, Bill took the brochures for the funeral homes and tossed them in the trash.

Such a kind man to look out for him and pass along the positive feedback. He hadn't needed those brochures anyway. Carl smiled, relishing in Bill's praise. "Yeah, I guess you're right, Bill. I did do good with that family, didn't I?"

"Hell yes! That was a wife, an ex-wife, *and* a girlfriend? And you walked in the middle of their bickering and just laid it on the line like a boss! Wait, what was it you said? 'I'm so sorry to inform you Mr. Samson didn't make it. But I am told his final words to our dedicated healthcare providers were, "Please tell my one true love that I will forever be in her heart." It's times like these, when the end has come, that you know the amazing power of love.' When they teared up and hugged, I mean, just wow!"

Carl grinned ear to ear. "Yeah, I heard it in a song this morning, driving in. It had a nice ring to it."

"Yeah it did! So don't beat yourself up over our future at D-MACS, OK? Things are going good for us, pal. Real good."

"Thanks, Bill. You're right. I just get kinda worried sometimes. But if you say things are good, then I'm good."

"Things are more than good, actually. I'm probably not supposed to say this, but, what the heck? If things keep going like they are, we're looking at a pretty nice bonus this year. But you didn't hear it from me!" Bill raised both hands in front of him to emphasize his attempt at plausible deniability.

Carl's smile grew even bigger. He was relieved to know things were going well and promised himself to never second guess Bill again. After all, he had never steered him wrong yet.

"Now, come on. I hear another ambulance pulling in. You want me to take it?"

"Are you kidding me? I got this, Bill. Oh, I got this!"

Walking away, Carl felt back on track. He was glad to have regained his purpose. If Bill was right, and he certainly was, D-MACS was doing better than ever.

TRUST... BUT VERIFY

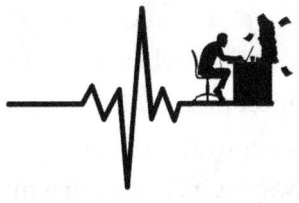

CHAPTER TEN

Harry was the master at navigating multiple conversations at once. Well ... he usually was. But, hey, even Babe Ruth struck out now and then. On his left side, Evan was excitedly discussing something going on with his work. But on his right side, two juiced up jokers were entangled in a war of words and using their drinks to punctuate each zinger. Harry wanted to pay more attention to Evan—he really did. He'd been in quite the state ever since he'd entered Houlihan's. But these two libated inebriates demanded his attention.

"You're crazy, you know it?" the first drunkard slurred, gesturing wildly with his glass (liquid sloshing) at his pal's torso. "This is ... this is ... what is this? This is absurdity, that's what this is."

Evan continued his own animated oration to Harry, obviously unaware of his uncle's auditory tug-of-war. "I can't support it and I just won't, you know what I mean?"

As if on cue, Harry subconsciously picked up on Evan's pause and grunted in the affirmative at the correct time. All the while, he was navigating his bar towel around the bar flies, sopping up their alcohol-infused exclamation points.

"I'm crazy? (Hiccup) What about you? I mean, you live with yer mom and ... and ... and you have the nerve to show up here tonight wearing—what is it yer wearing anyhow? Yellow? A yellow (hiccup) shirt? I mean, who wears yellow?" To emphasize his point, the boozer waved wildly around Houlihan's Hideaway, as if proving that his lush partner was alone in his color choice. As he continued waving around in a full three-hundred-and-sixty degrees, he knocked over a napkin dispenser and two laminated table tent cards advertising "Thursday TRIVIA!" and "BAIL BONDs FAST— Call NOW!" His remaining third of a glass of well-brand bourbon splashed on his partner's neon-yellow shirt.

Catching the tent cards in one hand, Harry tossed his saturated towel to the side and retrieved a dry towel from under the bar with his other hand in anticipation of more potable precipitation from the duo. At the same time, he managed to cast a glance at Evan and quickly interject a "Hell yeah! That's telling them, squirt!" before zeroing back in on the obnoxious duo.

"NOW LOOK WHAT YOU DID!" shouted the spirits-soaked sot to his drinking buddy. "Yer gonna ... yer gonna ... gon' buy me a new shirt! That's what yer gonna do, *bozo!*"

The two men grabbed each other's shirts and struggled with each other, glass breaking and liquid spilling, while Harry tried to intervene, all the while listening to Evan go on about *something*, oblivious to the melee next to him.

"Uh-huh. Yeah, that sounds like it would work," Harry

said over his shoulder to Evan as he nimbly settled both boozers back on their barstools, breaking up the argument.

"Thanks, Harry. I've never felt more alive! You're the best! I'm going to do it! I mean, I wasn't sure I was going to do it, because it's crazy, right? But sometimes you just gotta get in there and make your own destiny, you know? I mean, yeah! You don't think I'll get fired over this, do you? I mean, I guess they'd have to catch me first, and since the left hand doesn't know what the right hand is doing around there, I'd have a good chance. It's gotta be subtle and it's gotta be stealthy. And I know just how to do it. Thanks!"

And with that, Evan was gone.

Now, after closing, Harry cleaned up the bar in his nightly ritual of readying the business for its morning clientele. As he wiped down the tables and barstools with his towel, he couldn't stop thinking about Evan. He had never seen him so ... *confident*.

"He's a good kid, don't get me wrong," Harry told his reflection in the polished wood of the bar. "But confident? Nah, not our Evan. Wonder what's gotten into him?"

Harry had listened—albeit with a moderate amount of distraction from the drunken duo—to his ideas about how he was going to go into the office and do ... *something*. Harry had nodded and agreed but was, admittedly, not exactly sure what Evan was talking about.

Spraying the tables and barstools with cleaner, Harry continued to scrub off the night's revelry while straining to recall Evan's conversation.

"What was it? Quick something? Quiet something? Q-word. Q-word. What the hell was Evan talking about?

Why didn't I listen to him more closely?"

Scrubbing a stubborn stain on the barstool, Harry could not for the life of him figure out what he had encouraged him to do.

Well, I'm sure it isn't *too* out there. After all, it's Evan. Well, maybe it is a *little* out there? What was it Evan had been talking about?

"Quiet sabotage." That's what it was. Quiet sabotage.

Now what on earth could that mean to Evan?

Focusing his attention now on the floors, Harry worried Evan might be getting in over his head. He knew his nephew better than just about anyone. But Evan? And sabotage? Nah. I mean, could he? Nah.

As Harry peeled dried gum off of the underside of the bar (*Who chews gum in a bar?*), he grew worried. Not really knowing what Evan did for a living other than it involving healthcare, computers, and government agencies, it didn't sound to Harry like the wise move to "quiet sabotage" anything.

Harry calmed himself by singing "We're Not Gonna Take It" by Twisted Sister to amplify Evan's most recent defiant declaration. He then laughed to himself, imagining Evan wearing full gouache makeup and a comical blonde curly 80s wig and it made him feel better.

"The kid's gonna be OK," Harry said to the small pile of trash in the corner that he swept up into a dustbin.

"Yeah, the kid's gonna be just fine," Harry lied to himself as he let the 80s anthem of anarchy lull him away from his troubles. "Just fine."

It had been months (wait, had it been over a year?) since Dr. Thompkins had stepped foot into the D-MACS office building down the street from his own office. This branch housed the support service departments such as accounting, payroll, quality control ... and the panelists, among others. What in the world did these people do all day? As he stood on the sidewalk in front of the building, he stared in wonder at the multiple floors, unable to see the top floor from his vantage point near the front entrance.

As a physician, he understood research, peer reviews, and the need to deep dive into the science of the art of medicine. He understood patient assessments and the "laying of hands" on the sick to elicit the secrets to better health. But the roles like "administration" or "human resources" were too ethereal for him to comprehend. How did they fill a whole business day? They probably endured endless meetings, sometimes meeting to decide what they would need to meet about. He laughed, thinking about it. "Meeting to meet about a meeting—hah!"

He shook his head. That sounded about right when it came to a bureaucratic entity like D-MACS. He felt thankful his role was more tangible and he could clearly understand his role. Except for this assignment. His smile evaporated. Although he understood the task at hand, it didn't ease his sense of dread of meeting with ... what was his name again? Dr. Thompkins fumbled around in his pants pockets, then his jacket pockets, finally locating the crumpled piece of paper onto which he had jotted down in his almost illegible handwriting:

Theodore Butler

What's at Stake
URGENT

Reading the handwritten note, he was reminded of the phone conversation with Samantha and felt troubled by the request. She had changed the rules midstream, and he couldn't help wondering if she had anything to do with the obituary he had received ... and the suspicious death of his colleague. What would she do if this Theodore didn't "straighten up and fly right," as she phrased it. And, more importantly, what would happen to *him* if he weren't able to convince Theodore of "what's at stake." While standing outside the building, considering how he would handle this task, he was slightly bumped by a hurried passerby.

Startled, Dr. Thompkins formed his most disapproving sneer to be targeted at his jostler to show his disdain for such carelessness. He turned.

"Oh, my goodness, I am so sorry sir—I was in a hurry and wasn't paying attention. Oh, hey! Dr. Thompkins! Are you OK? What are you doing down here? I was just headed back in." He gestured toward the D-MACS building. "I'm sorry again, sir."

Dr. Thompkins stared at Evan, taking a few seconds to recognize the D-MACS panelist ... then smiling at him in an attempt to be reassuring and forgiving.

"Quite all right, young man. I bet you're just in a hurry to get back to some good, hard work, aren't you?" Dr. Thompkins said with a wink. In fact, I'm on my way to see your team and touch base with the troops. Shall we go up together?"

Evan's eyes widened though Dr. Thompkins noted the quick change to a neutral expression.

"Of course, Dr. Thompkins! I know everyone will be really honored to have you up on the floor." Evan said, cheeks turning red. "And who knows? Maybe we'll log you in as a guest panelist!" His follow-up laugh was a little too jolly.

"Watch out, Evan! I just might take you up on that!" Dr. Thompkins felt just as awkward as Evan seemed to be. They both laughed loudly at his rejoinder, however, with Dr. Thompkins hoping his at least sounded natural.

Together, they entered the government office building and flashed their D-MACS badges at the security guard on their way to the bank of elevators. Waiting for the elevator, they attempted to discuss the weather, the score of the game last night, and a documentary Evan had recently watched in which he had learned that dolphins have no sense of smell.

"Can't smell a thing, huh? Well, how about that?" Dr. Thompkins hoped his tortured grin conveyed interest instead of his true feelings. He silently kicked himself for failing to just pick up the phone and call Theo instead of implementing this torturous exercise in civility and socializing.

As they entered the elevator, several D-MACS employees filed in with them.

"How're you doing, Frank?"

"Another day in paradise. How about you?"

"Well, any day above ground is a good day, so can't complain. How 'bout you, Pam?"

"Overworked and underpaid."

Dr. Thompkins was fascinated by the level of their mindless dribble. Solitude was so much more preferable.

During the elevator ride, several employees entered and

exited on different floors, each with variations on a theme of inane greetings.

"If I were any better, they'd have to take me out and shoot me."

"Living the dream!"

Dr. Thompkins sent up a silent prayer of thanks as the elevator finally reached Evan's floor.

As soon as the two exited, however, Dr. Thompkins immediately regretted leaving the sanctuary of the elevator and made a mental note to never do this again.

"Hi! I'm Murray!"

Peg had never met the old man who stood in the lobby and was curious as to the animation among her co-workers this morning. With his wiry, wind-tussled hair and curmudgeonly attire, she thought he might be a tenured professor who had gotten off on the wrong floor. Or maybe he was somebody's grandfather, stopping in to wish someone a happy birthday? As she watched Murray hold him in a captive audience, she could tell the gentleman was obviously trying to get away, but didn't know how to navigate his way out of the verbal sleeper hold that only Murray knew how to wield. She decided to approach and rescue if needed. No one deserved that type of punishment, right?

"So this girl, right, she goes out with me two, wait, no, three times and then decides to try to pull the old 'I have to tend to my sick aunt' routine with the old Murr? I say, 'No way, lady—it's your loss, not mine. Not mine.' I mean, am I right, Doc? Am I right? So I am currently 'single and ready to mingle' as they say. You don't happen to know any eligible—"

"I'm so sorry to interrupt," interrupted Peg, as panic filled the old man's eyes. "But I'm Peg, I work here for D-MACS. And you are?" She extended her hand and pulled the man away from the Murr-a-caine.

"Oh, why I'm Dr. Harold Thompkins," he said, grabbing onto her hand as if he were clutching onto a life preserver.

Walking away from Murray's scowl and "Hey! We were talkin'," Dr. Thompkins patted Peg's arm.

"Thank you, thank you, thank you, dear lady. What, exactly, was that?" Dr. Thompkins gave a full-body shiver.

"Well, sir, that was Murray, and I think he's harmless enough. He tends to have a way, though, doesn't he? Anyway, are you looking for someone? Are you lost?"

"No, no, no. It's great to make your acquaintance. I'm actually one of the directors here at D-MACS. I don't come to this floor often, though I guess I should. I work down the street in our other office building, and I thought I should come down and check on the troops, as it were. Are you one of the panelists here?"

As Peg opened her mouth to respond, she saw Evan over Dr. Thompkins's shoulder trying to get her attention. She bobbed her head, indicating she'd seen him, and in response he tipped his head toward the breakroom before disappearing into it.

"Um, yes, yes I am one of the panelists here at D-MACS. I recently got hired on and, although I've still got a lot to learn, I am really enjoying the job. I apologize, but I'm running late for a meeting … was there someone you were specifically wanting to meet with?"

"Well, actually, yes. I was wondering if Theodore Butler is available?" Dr. Thompkins peered around the office at the rows and rows of cubicles, and Peg caught his wrinkled-nose expression before his face cleared again.

The poor man seemed overwhelmed, Peg thought. "Oh sure, sure. Theo is around here … um … somewhere …" Peg quickly scanned over and around the various cubicles and finally saw Theo speaking with Keisha, Joanna, Tina, and Charlene down the hall.

"There he is, sir. Right this way."

Peg guided Dr. Thompkins through the maze of cubicles toward Theo.

As they approached, Theo changed his tone into something deeper and slightly condescending. Peg pursed her lips.

"So, I fully expect to see an increase in your productivity immediately. Is that clear? I said, is that clear, ladies?"

Peg almost expected him to click his heels. Keisha, Joanna, Tina, and Charlene, meanwhile, exchanged a glance and burst out into spontaneous laughter.

"Good one, Theo." Keisha replied.

"Yes sir! Right away, sir!" Joanna gave a smart salute.

"Say what?" Tina interjected, hands on hips.

"You better check yourself, Theo, before you—" Charlene caught sight of them. "Oh, hi." She extended her hand to Dr. Thompkins as they pulled up next to them.

Peg took the opportunity to draw Dr. Thompkins's attention with a quick introduction to Theo and a goodbye before doubling back to the breakroom.

Dr. Thompkins quickly shook Theo's hand before formally introducing himself to the ladies.

"Hello, hello. I'm Dr. Thompkins, one of the medical directors here at D-MACS. It's my pleasure to meet each of you."

He proceeded to exchange pleasantries with each of them before turning back to Theo.

"I met you after the last update conference, Dr. Thompkins. But you probably don't remember me."

Dr. Thompkins felt relief that Peg had pointed out the shift supervisor to him as he had no idea who he was. "Of course I remember you, young Theodore! It's terrific to see you again. As I understand it, you're the task master of this well-oiled machine up here, correct? What a great job you are doing!"

Keisha, Joanna, Tina, and Charlene rolled their eyes in unison and filed off toward their individual cubicles in perfect synchrony. Theo was left alone with the director.

"Actually, Theodore, it is you specifically I am here to see. Could I steal a moment of your time to discuss something? In private perhaps?"

Theo shifted weight from one foot to the other. And wiped his palms against his pants. "Of course, um, sure. Let's see, how about we use the conference room over here?" Theo pointed to the floor-to-ceiling glass room in the middle of the floor, surrounded by panelists' cubicles.

Dr. Thompkins eyed the glass-walled room and immediately dismissed this offering as being too visually public for his liking. "Well, actually, how about your office?"

Um, well, um, sure. No problem. Come this way." Massaging his neck, Theo led the way through the maze of cubicles to his office, which was located in a darkened back hallway away from the main work area.

Dr. Thompkins felt he should be making small talk but honestly had no idea what to say. He silently followed Theo into the room as Theo flicked on the light. He waited as Theo closed the door and moved over to his desk. Rather than take a seat, Theo stood there and looked inquisitively at him.

Holding in a sigh, Dr. Thompkins took initiative. The poor boy seemed woefully inept. "Please, please, have a seat, young Theodore. Please." Dr. Thompkins nodded toward Theo's office chair as he perched on a tattered upholstered chair next to the desk.

Theo slowly sat down behind his desk, his lips pressed together, eyebrows furrowed.

"Theo. Can I call you Theo?"

Theo nodded.

"Yes? Thank you. Theo, have you heard of Dr. Stephen Hawking?"

"Um, yes?"

"I have always been fascinated by his writings and theories on black holes. Simply fascinating stuff. He famously once said something along the lines of 'Intelligence is the ability to adapt to change.' I've always subscribed to the same school of thought. The ability to adapt to change."

He held out his hands, palm side up. "On the one hand, we have incredibly smart *academic* people who can take tests well and achieve a high level of post-graduate work but wouldn't be able to make a peanut butter sandwich without an instructional manual. You know what I am saying?"

Theo shook his head then quickly nodded, eyebrows puckered.

"And on the other hand, we have incredibly smart *emotionally* intelligent people who can run Fortune 500 companies ... but can't add two and two together. Right?"

This time, no movement from Theo.

Dr. Thompkins rapped his knuckles against his knee. "But intelligence, *true* intelligence, to me, is the ability to combine the two and pivot when needed. To adapt to change."

To make his point, he clasped his hands together in front of himself.

"Adaptability. That takes true intelligence. Book smarts and street smarts, as they say. It's truly an amazing thing to see. And those who have this gift are wondrous creatures who walk among the common people in our society."

Theo stared at him with vacuous eyes and squirmed in his seat.

As Dr. Thompkins sized up Theo, he felt sorry for him, a simple-minded supervisor who obviously struggled to follow the logic of his preamble. He decided to cut to the chase for the wilting flower before him.

"You, young Theodore, are lacking the cognition and discernment needed at this pivotal time. And, as such, your inability to adapt to change is deleterious to our mission."

Blinking at Dr. Thompkins, Theo opened his mouth then closed it.

Seeing the puzzlement in Theo's eyes, Dr. Thompkins was reminded of the thousands of times he had delivered bad news to patients using medical jargon that was miles over their heads. They would continue to optimistically smile at him, despite telling them that they were actively dying. He realized quickly of the need to "dumb it down" for Theo as he had to do for numerous terminal patients of the past.

"Word has gotten back to upper admin that your panelists are showing signs of not supporting Status Quotient. The Code Orange of recent, involving our local celebrity chef, was not met with the unquestioning confidence we expect and require. Correct?"

It took a moment before Theo's eyes widened, and a slow flush colored his cheeks. Giving a short nod, he slumped in his seat. Then his face cleared momentarily, and he straightened a bit. "Yeah, but—"

"No 'buts,' Theo." Dr. Thompkins rose to his feet so as to emphasize the gravity of the situation. "I need to know you understand what's at stake here." He leaned forward, bracing his hands against the desktop. "As D-MACS pivots to this new variable, we need to have one hundred percent confidence that you are on board in order for the beta testing to be successful. Are you on board?"

Theo swallowed, Adam's apple bobbing. "Yes, sir, of course I am. You don't need to worry about ol' Theo. I'm your guy. I'll get these dissenters in line, you betcha."

"Good, good. I'm glad to hear this, young Theodore. I had a feeling I could count on you." Dr. Thompkins did his best to smile a vote of confidence, an outright lie.

Fortunately, Theo didn't appear to detect the insincerity.

"How about I give you a call in a week or so? You know, just to touch base and ensure we are all heading in the right direction. Sound good?"

Theo stood and shook Dr. Thompkins' outstretched

hand. "Of course, sir, that would be just swell. I'm on it!"

Dr. Thompkins released Theo's weak handshake. There wasn't any more he could offer to the shift supervisor that would be of benefit. He thanked him and told him he would see himself out.

As Dr. Thompkins meandered through the rows of cubicles, he took the time to speak with a few of the panelists to encourage them as best he could.

"The job you are doing, collectively, is changing the course of healthcare for the future. Never forget that!"

"Each chart you review is an important piece of this puzzle!"

"Because of each of you, we are making a real difference in the lives of our patients. Thank you!"

The panelists were cordial enough to him, but a collective sigh of relief was palpable when Dr. Thompkins finally made his way to the elevator. His own joined them as the doors shut behind him. No, this job wasn't turning out as expected.

Evan waited in the breakroom as Peg got her coffee and took a seat across from him. As the steam rose from Peg's Hello Kitty coffee cup, he saw the worry on her face and wondered where her concern stemmed from.

Hoping he was making the right choice, he leaned forward and pointed out the breakroom door. "Did you see that, Peg?" Evan whispered in a hoarse voice while confirming no one else was in the breakroom. "Did you? Dr. Thompkins himself? Here! On *our* floor! I mean, what the heck."

"I don't understand. Why does it upset you, Evan?" Peg's forehead bunched up.

Evan hesitated to respond. How much should he share with her? He recognized Peg was a perceptive, quick learner. He thought she could help him with his plan. She certainly seemed eager to help. As he took a sip of his coffee, he made his decision.

"Well, I guess it's alright to share with you. You promise not to discuss this with anyone?"

Peg nodded and leaned in.

Evan shared his recent visit to Dr. Thompkins, his own misgivings about the direction D-MACS was taking with Status Quotient … and his idea on how to subvert the whole new initiative. As Evan described in detail to Peg his plan, her face reflected a myriad of emotions, ranging from surprise to worry and ending with … excitement? Partnering with Peg on this would likely be an adventure all on its own, way outside his comfort zone. But, together, they just might be able to pull off his "quiet sabotage."

One patient chart at a time.

SMOKE 'EM IF YA GOT 'EM

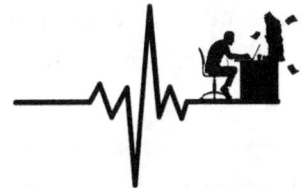

CHAPTER ELEVEN

Frank Turzanski hated his life. No. That's not the word. Despised. Yes, despised. Staring out his office window overlooking the factory floor, sipping Wild Turkey out of a Styrofoam coffee cup, he couldn't help but think of how best to atone for his sins. And sins, he had aplenty. Watching the factory workers assemble the frames of midsize SUVs, he tried to figure out how his life had gotten to this point. Surely it wasn't too late to turn it all around, was it? At sixty-two, his efforts to convince himself that a glimmer of hope remained in his tiresome life grew dimmer and dimmer each day. "How did I get here?" he mused, sipping from his cup. Looking around his office to emphasize to himself his wonderment of self-direction, he happened to see the black-and-white picture of his former glory days hanging over his desk, and a faint smile appeared on his face for the first time in weeks.

As a semi-pro wrestler with Extreme Wrestling Entertainment, he recalled some of the best days of his life on the circuit. Frank "The Tank" Turzanski was a formidable opponent and always gave the fans their money's worth when he was in the ring. With his signature move encouraged by the crowd, they could be counted on to chant "Tank him! Tank him! Tank him!" in a fevered frenzy. Frank would then run full force, bouncing against the ropes and become "The Tank." With his head down, he would run full force into his opponent like a tank, headbutting him into oblivion.

After three or four years of his trademark move, he had a small following. He was able to sell merchandise after matches, such as sequined capes and T-shirts with his likeness on them and *"Tank Him!"* emblazoned underneath. He made a decent living out of it and felt like life couldn't get any better. His wife, Betty, manned the merchandise booth and traveled with him in their RV on the East Coast circuit, most matches being held in high school gyms and local YMCAs. Extreme Wrestling Entertainment, LLC, paid fairly well and encouraged the entrepreneurial spirit of each of the wrestlers. They eked out a living and enjoyed the time as best as they could.

Then came the neck and back pain.

After years of ramming his head into two hundred-and-fifty-pound grown-men's torsos, his intervertebral disks began herniating and causing excruciating pain. Doctors were expensive and surgery was out of the question, forcing Frank to retire from wrestling and find gainful employment elsewhere. Betty, who thought touring the country with a semi-pro wrestler was fun and exciting, quickly became disenchanted with Frank "The Tank" working as a line foreman at a car manufacturing plant. Turned out, she loved the wrestler, hated the man.

The divorce cost him dearly. Betty moved on with Billy "The Bulldozer" Bentley, taking the RV with her. They had never made time for children, and Frank never remarried, thinking Betty would eventually tire of the glamour and glitz of the local wrestling circuit and come back to him. Twenty-three years later, Frank still carried a torch for Betty that had yet to be extinguished, no matter how much Wild Turkey he consumed to douse the flames. He eventually became married to his job, pulling whatever shifts were needed to help pay the alimony payments to Betty.

As he looked over the factory line, Frank finally realized his life was tiresome and insignificant. And he despised his life.

Raising the coffee cup of bourbon to his lips, he heard the alarms blare from the factory floor. He placed his cup on his desk to make his way down to the line. It was not unusual to have a safety alarm sound on the assembly line as any potential safety violation caused an immediate shut down of the entire line in accordance with OSHA standards. Usually it was caused by a faulty placement of a bolt here or a loose nut there. Only the line foreman could reset the line and disable the alarm after investigating the source of violation.

Seeing one of the worker's legs pinned under the car, however, prompted Frank to immediately run toward the scene. It had been years since any injuries had occurred on the factory floor. A sign stating "557 DAYS—NO WORKPLACE INJURIES" was located on the wall immediately over Frank's head as he approached the downed car frame, shouts and screams surrounding him.

"Dammit." Frank said as he saw the scene before him.

Approximately two years ago, Frank was coerced to hire undocumented immigrants by upper management. No. That wasn't the word. Forced. Yes, *forced*. With low pay, and even lower benefits, getting enough factory workers was difficult, and Frank found himself having to outsource factory linemen to these undocumented workers. He learned some key words to communicate with them, and they served him well as they were punctual, hard workers, and never complained—at least not to him. Seeing Jose Gonzales pinned under the car, Frank's mind immediately went to the paperwork that would ensue, some of which would require regulatory oversight inquiries, including hiring practices. Not wanting to get gummed down by the red tape, Frank jumped into action.

Correction: Frank "The Tank" jumped into action.

Frank grabbed the side of the car frame, which had somehow dislodged from the assembly line joists, and lifted it as if he were back on the Extreme Wrestling Entertainment circuit, fully expecting to hear cheers from his fans.

Instead, he heard the loud pop in his back and then everything went black. Frank "The Tank" was down, and it looked like this time it was for the final count.

Ambulance #37 pulled up to the automobile manufacturing facility as directed by dispatch, after the 9-1-1 call was placed by the associate foreman. As they were winding through the factory floor with their stretcher and medical tackle boxes, Terrell and Carlos were deep into their betting already.

"Fifty dollars?" Terrell's eyebrows rose. "You're crazy, man. I ain't bettin' no fifty dollars on this one."

Carlos shot a goading smile at Terrell. "What? You scared? I'm telling you. This is a wasted call. First off, look around. Everyone here is either undocumented or minimum wage. We ain't goin' to Regional Gen—we're too close to it. And we ain't hittin' the lights. C'mon. If you think I'm lyin', put your money where your mouth is."

Terrell gazed around the factory. Carlos was spot on with his quick assessment. Maybe he'd taught his protege well—perhaps even a little too well. As they approached the crowd of onlookers and factory workers, Terrell decided to boost his partner's spirit a little. "All right. Fifty dollars. But it's gotta be no lights, no siren, and *two* hospitals away. Two."

"Two? Shit, man. Hmmm, OK. " The EMTs quickly shook hands to confirm the bet.

Terrell expertly navigated the gurney into the crowd, grabbed his gear off its surface, and assessed the chaotic scene. Several Hispanic factory workers were crowded around an older man who, to Terrell's surprise, had not been involved in any type of machinery-caused accident. A few feet away from him, more workers were gathered around an Hispanic man who was sitting upright, next to a partially assembled car. He was smiling and rubbing his legs, with no indication of any injury.

Terrell and Carlos immediately focused their attention on the older man. Working together with effortless synchrony, they barely said a word as they quickly and methodically provided resuscitative assistance to "The Tank". Once they got him stabilized, Terrell called it in.

"Dispatch, this is Shaver. We got a 62-year-old white male who had a syncopal episode of unknown origin. Presents as a spinal cord injury of some fashion as he is unable to move and has no sensation from the nipple line down. We have already intubated to protect his airway. He's satting 98 percent on 100 percent O2. Heart rate 84. BP is stable at 148/86. We're about to load him up and need to know where you'd like for us to deliver. Over."

As they placed the patient on the stretcher, Carlos gave Terrell an up-nod. "I'm telling you, ain't no ways we're heading to Rege Gen, Terrell. Ain't no ways."

Terrell eyed the patient as he bagged him. Morbidly obese. Hypertension. Reeked of alcohol (*It's only nine thirty in the morning, for crying out loud!*). Lately, patients in worse condition than this were relegated to going to the hospital furthest away. He knew Carlos was right. This poor guy was going to get the worst chance, thanks to D-MACS.

No one was more surprised than Terrell when dispatch instructed them to immediately take him to Regional General for immediate treatment.

Carlos stared at Terrell, then the patient, then back at Terrell and shook his head in disbelief. "What? What's going on with dispatch, huh? I mean, good for this guy, but damn. I don't get it."

As they pushed the loaded stretcher back to Ambulance #37, Carlos wore an expression of disappointment and muttered about sending the money later. Once the patient was loaded, Carlos situated himself in the back of the truck to continue ventilating the intubated patient while Terrell hustled around to the driver's seat.

After firing the engine, he made a quick exit, lights flashing and sirens wailing. Terrell was glad as he made a beeline toward the nearest hospital. Finally, someone getting help. "Good for you, man. Good for you."

Evan made his way around the cubicles, nodding secret thanks to his fellow panelists who had successfully adjusted the score for the sixty-two-year-old spinal cord injury. Frank Turzanski was Evan's first experiment in beating the system. He had a less-than-optimal health score rating and an even worse Status Quotient. Frank had not paid his taxes in, well, had never paid income taxes that could be found. Was not a member of any charitable organizations. Was behind on his alimony payments. Nearing retirement age, he showed no signs of having made any social contributions in the past, present, nor likely in the future. In fact, Frank owed his life to having his chart reviewed by Evan and his mishmash cohort of like-minded revolutionaries. With the overwhelming consensus of scores being manually manipulated by the majority of panelists, Frank was able to be stabilized and receive dexamethasone in a timely manner, treating his spinal cord compression and eventually regaining movement and sensation.

As Evan was rounding the cubicles, giving silent signs of appreciation to Keisha, Joanna, Tina, and Charlene, Theo rounded the corner. Evan immediately made his way back to his own cubicle before being seen.

Murray was waiting at Evan's desk. He narrowed his eyes. "What are you up to, Putz?"

Evan had intentionally left Murray out of the loop in order to keep his plan intact and, hopefully, unnoticed by Theo or others.

"Um, you know, just stretching my legs. I read somewhere that you should walk every hour to prevent blood clots. Keeps me healthy, y'know, Murr?"

"You're seriously an idiot, you know that? Do you believe everything you read, dummy? Why don't you just get back to your work and stop flitting around the office like a freakin' butterfly?" To elaborate on this, Murray flapped his hands.

"You got it, Murr. Thanks for keeping me focused." Evan did his best to disengage Murray and not give him any more reason to ask questions or be too inquisitive. "Here I go, back to my computer. You should probably get to work too."

For emphasis, Evan flapped his hands, eliciting a snort from Murray and a head shake of disapproval.

"What a putz you are."

Evan logged on to his station and considered what he had just accomplished. He had enough experience to know what scores would get flagged and which would not. Also, he had calculated correctly how many panelists were needed to successfully combat the score manipulation created by Status Quotient. Not too many, not too few. Not too high, not too low. Just right. Giving Murray time to situate himself at his own desk, he confirmed again to himself the wise decision to not involve him in this covert scoring plan. Now, how to keep Theo from getting wind of anything? Evan was not exactly sure how much oversight the role of shift supervisor had in each reviewed case and was therefore limited in his estimation of how much or how soon Theo would know.

All Theo appeared to do was walk around ensuring everyone was present and accounted for and, well, that was about it. Evan was not sure what type of reports the shift supervisor had or even if Theo paid attention to any of them.

He *did* know the scoring of each case was tabulated and available for each panelist to review. The consolidated feedback response was blinded at Evan's level, only showing how many panelists had scored a chart, what the average score was for the case, what the highest and lowest scores were, and what the final outcome was. Evan decided to pull up the numbers to see how the numbers fared across the group. After verifying that Murray was busy on his phone, he pulled up the chart.

Though the bell curve was there, it was less pronounced than he would have liked. As expected, several panelists had scored higher than Evan and his group. However, Evan had correctly selected the right number of panelists to join him on his crusade to move the number back toward center and provide a lowered overall score. Staring at the screen, Evan felt confident that no one of Theo's level would raise an eyebrow at this grouping of scores. He minimized the screen moments before Theo came walking in his direction.

Peg was skulking in the background, obviously anxious about Theo's increased pace beelining toward Evan's cubicle. They had both planned to watch for Theo, sharing a concern that he might be smarter than they had given him credit for. Evan buried his face in his computer, becoming as busy as he could possibly look.

"Can I interrupt you for a second?" Theo stated, contrived authority ringing in his tone. "Something has come up, and I think you know what I'm talking about."

Pulse racing, Evan turned around to face him and was surprised to see Theo had his back to him.

He was talking to Murray!

"Yeah, Theo … what's up, my man?" Murray fumbled to put his phone away but not before Theo pointed to it and cleared his throat.

"Let's go talk in my office, shall we?"

Evan relaxed his shoulders as Theo led Murray away. As soon as they disappeared, Peg popped her head in, lips turned up in a relieved smile. Evan motioned with his eyes toward the breakroom, to which Peg gave a slight nod before heading away.

Evan waited two minutes, then joined her.

Peg stood at the counter near the coffee station. "Oh. My. God," she said under her breath as she filled her coffee cup. "That was scary, wasn't it?" She nudged him. "I thought for sure he was coming to talk to you!"

Evan did his best to act nonchalant. "Oh, that? Nah, it's fine. We got this. We were careful enough for Theo not to catch on to anything."

"Oh, totally. I mean, nothing to it, right?" She pushed the carafe toward him.

"Uh, yeah, so I just wanted to say I reviewed the CFR, and the bell curve looks perfect. I didn't see anything that would send up a red flag."

"Oh, that's good to know." Peg blew on her coffee for a few seconds before taking a sip, eyeing him over the rim. She reached out to lean on the counter, misjudging her distance by mere inches. She stumbled slightly in her misstep, spilling coffee in her wake. She quickly grabbed the closest handtowel to clean up her mess.

Evan, not knowing what to do, turned his back to Peg to pour himself a cup of coffee and let on that he didn't see her stumble and add to her embarrassment. As he did so, he noticed his hands shaking and did not want her to see his own nervousness. He set down the carafe and faced her again, willing his hand to hold steady.

He took a calming breath. "And this is the right thing to do, Peg. Right? I feel it. This is our way of fighting the system, in a way. I don't know. I mean, whatever." Evan, again, did his best to act cool, calm, and collected. As he brought his coffee cup to his lips, his shaking hands belied his nerves.

Peg, without hesitating, reached her hand out to Evan's, steadying his shaking coffee cup before its contents would slosh out.

"It *is* the right thing, Evan. It truly is. And I think it is wonderful that you came up with this. I'm with you. You are so smart and I admire you so much for this. Yes. It is a way to fight the system. A great way. Ever since I started here, I've felt somewhat conflicted about what we're doing. It didn't take long to see how the system is coerced and rigged against most people. Originally, I thought I was truly helping people, but then something felt off. And then, with this Status Quotient thing, it became glaringly obvious the system is only out for one thing. To save a buck. But now you've given me hope. You've given hope to all of us who you have asked to help. Thank you, Evan."

Evan's hands had stopped shaking, but he wasn't ready for her to let go yet.

Apparently, neither was Peg. She gave him a reassuring squeeze and made no move to pull away.

Harry polished the bar while listening to the soused boozer in front of him, waiting for his cue to offer up agreement or sympathy, whatever the tone and cadence called for.

"It's like, I dunno, it's like she used me for the best years of my life and then just tossed me to the curb like a pile of trash. It ain't fair, I tells ya. It just ain't fair!"

Harry had long ago stopped needing to pay attention to the soliloquies offered up by the lone actors who spent their time and money on barstools. Now, take your typical guy who had been dumped by his wife/girlfriend/mistress. His paraverbal tell-tales would be somewhat higher in pitch and accompanied by tears and nose blowing. The guy could be speaking Hindu for all Harry cared. It was the same every time. Harry dubbed these "sad sacks" as they were blindsided and had little to do with the ousting.

But if the lamenter had more of a responsibility and ownership in the rejection, his voice would be somewhat more defensive and louder, typically with more hand motions. More anger, less hurt. These types were known in Harry's dictionary as "the comeuppance" as they were, well, getting what they deserved.

Harry's favorite, hands down, however, was the griever who had left his spouse for another woman, only to be rejected by the other woman, and now he wanted to reconcile with his wife. Only to be rejected by her as well. Harry called these "double dumps" and was fascinated by the uniformity of their stories. Unfortunately for Harry, this was not one of those.

This was your dime-a-dozen sob stories offered up by a "sad sack," the most common and, for Harry, the most pitiful. These poor guys were rather clueless as to what happened to them and were helpless as to how to handle their lives going forth. So they looked to Harry for comfort, consolation, counseling … and cocktails.

Sensing his cue, Harry offered up a "That is just terrible, man" coupled with a "That just isn't fair." The sad sack let out one final wail of anguish and collapsed on the bar. So as to not disturb the other customers, this was Harry's next cue to go around the bar with a fresh drink, compliments of Houlihan's Hideaway, and lead the guy to a booth out of earshot of the rest of the bar.

"There, there. Here you go, have one on the house, friend."

Sniffing and sipping, the cries would invariably lessen, leaving the dejected and despondent soon-to-be divorcee to his thoughts and soon-to-be-empty glass.

Walking back to his station behind the bar, Harry smiled as Evan came bounding through the door toward the bar.

"Well, there is a happy guy if ever I did see one!" Harry said to him, giving him a quick hug and offering a libation. "What will it be?"

"Your choice, Harry. I'm celebrating!"

"Let us celebrate the occasion with beer and words of cheer," Harry offered up, brow wrinkled as he tried to remember one of his favorite quotes. "It's so good to see that smile! What, exactly, are we celebrating?" Harry asked as he placed Evan's icy mug of frothy beer in front of him.

"It worked, Harry! It actually worked! And I tell ya, I just got to thank you for helping me out. I really appreciate your advice the other night." Evan beamed at his uncle.

"Well, you know, I've never let you down before, Squirt." Harry still was clueless as to how he had guided Evan, but took the offered credit, nonetheless.

"I went in there and, well, I don't know—something just came over me, and I had this overwhelming sense of calm and confidence. And I knew just what to do and just who to ask to help, and it worked, Harry!" Evan lifted his glass and offered up cheers.

"And then my shift supervisor came over toward me, and I thought the jig was up, honest to God I did Harry. My stomach turned to knots and I felt this heat coming over me, and lo and behold, he was coming to get on to a guy who works in my area for spending too much time on his phone instead of working. Oh, but, I dunno, I felt like even if he were coming to fire me or something, it would have been worth it. But it worked, it worked like clockwork, and I feel like I have a purpose now. So, here's to you, Harry!" Evan toasted him again, taking another large sip of his ale.

"So, what's next?" Harry asked as he gathered some used glasses and began the process of cleaning them and placing them away.

Evan took another sip and took a few seconds before responding.

"Well, I'm not really sure at this point. I guess I want to make sure this plan can work without raising any eyebrows, you know? But I gotta tell you, so far I feel good about it. And the group I put together is all on the same page, and it just feels really, really good. And there's this girl, Peg, who seems to really get me." A bigger smile appeared on Evan's face, and his cheeks reddened at the mention of her name.

Harry perked up. He had been wanting for years to hear Evan say someone's—*anyone's*—name. He had chalked him up as being too shy or maybe too tied to his work for anything else. Seeing Evan blush gave Harry new hope.

"Peg, huh? I haven't heard you mention a 'Peg' before, Squirt." Harry did his best to not seem too inquisitive, so he focused on restocking olives, lemons, and limes.

Evan cleared his throat. "Oh, Peg? She's just someone in my office I work with. That's all. She's nice."

Harry smiled at Evan.

"Stop it, Harry. She's a nice person, and that's it. OK? Drop it."

Harry knew when to push and when to retreat. He retreated.

"Sure thing. Want another?" Harry pointed to Evan's empty glass.

"Nah, I need to get home. I just wanted to stop in and thank you for supporting me and helping me out. I really appreciate everything you do for me, Harry."

"My pleasure. I'm proud of you, I really am. I know you're doing big things. Important things. And I'm proud of the difference you are making."

Evan beamed at him, then made his exit. As he did, Harry made sure to sing the theme song of *The Love Boat* loud enough for him to hear.

With a backhanded wave, Evan kept going.

WHEN IT RAINS, IT REALLY POURS

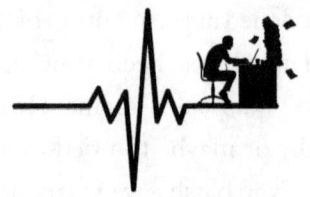

CHAPTER TWELVE

"Something's off here," Samantha muttered as she reviewed the latest D-MACS numbers. Earl had requested a financial review meeting for two o'clock, wanting to look over the most recent postings for the beta testing site. After a somewhat substantial few weeks of positive results, the numbers had shown an abrupt change. She felt confident in her approach to Dr. Thompkins and was sure he had gotten the message loud and clear of what was expected. But numbers didn't lie. It was as if not only the new initiative was not working, but progress made over the past year or two were erased as well. "This can't be." Samantha fumed. "This can't be."

Pursing her lips, she tried to consider what to do. Picking up the phone, she made a call to her source at Regional General to find out if her suspicions were right.

"Bill here."

"Hey, Bill, this is Sam. I haven't checked in with you recently and wanted to see if things were still 'slow and steady,' so to speak."

Bill Wilson cleared his throat and paused. Just when she was about to ask if everything was alright, he broke his silence.

"Well, Ms. McAllister, I'm going to lay my cards on the table. To be perfectly honest, we're drowning down here. Over the last couple of weeks, the floodgates have opened up, and we're bursting at the seams."

"We've got a full house and our ER is overflowing, with ambulances getting diverted to other facilities because we're out of room. Our doctors are raising hell, and I don't have a good answer for them. Seems like something has broken, and our staff's patience is running thin. Any insight or good news?"

Something like a creaking chair sounded in the background. She shifted in her own seat and tapped her pen on the desktop, thinking.

His voice interrupted. "Hello? Ms. McAllister? Did I lose you? Hello?"

"I'm here. Just trying to get my thoughts together. I appreciate your candidness. I really do. Do you have a sense of when the 'floodgates' opened on your end?"

"Well, let's see. Just gotta pull up my spread sheet, here." Bill made a "hmm" noise and after a moment, he said, "Looks like, well, yeah. Roughly about two, two and a half weeks ago. So, starting on the twelfth—and the patient numbers have held steady or increased even more ever since. I'm not sure what is going on, but we need some help, ma'am."

As he gave her his numbers, she compared her reports with his and a realization hit her. She decided to end the call.

"Thanks, Bill. I'm sorry for how busy it's been. I've got a

feeling it'll get back to normal. Let me make a few calls. Talk to you later." *Click*.

Samantha felt the heat of anger rise up in her—her previous messaging to the medical director of D-MACS must have been quickly forgotten, and he needed a more stern reminder. As she considered her options, she remembered her meeting with the CEO was quickly approaching. She'd need to put a spin on it to avoid any undue speculation or unwanted input. She just needed more time to get all the players back in line. In the meantime, she adjusted the timeframe for the data points that she would review with Earl so as to not alert him to any suspicions. She skewed the data in her favor, keeping the trendline going in the positive direction, knowing the CEO would not dive too deep in the weeds, and most likely would be satisfied with a glowing summary filled with optimism and continued success.

But Samantha would know. And so would Dr. Thompkins this evening. While she wasn't sure exactly what she would do yet, she was confident the solution would appear to her, as it always did. She had a knack for getting her way, and no aging physician was going to deter her success. She'd given him a "soft" warning last time. Perhaps it was time to let him know that she meant business. As she finalized her report and summary, printing the necessary number of copies, inspiration struck.

She let out a small laugh. "Yes. That would do it." With a smug smile, she congratulated herself for creating a plan so quickly. This was just a speed bump of inconvenience. Just a slight detour in her well-crafted roadmap to success. As she thought more about her plan, her anger dissipated and her confidence returned. "That will most definitely do it."

After Samantha gathered her reports together, she glanced at herself in the small mirror hanging on the wall nearest her door, ensuring that every hair was in place before heading to Earl Yarborough's office. She smiled at herself and gave a self-congratulatory wink.

"You got this!" she said. As satisfied as she was with her reports, she was even happier with her plan to get the message to Dr. Thompkins in a loud and clear manner. She did her best to look sad, wrinkling her brow and pouting in the mirror. "Poor guy. He won't know what hit him." Her devious laugh surprised her. After closing her office door, she walked toward the CEO's office.

"It's good to be me," Samantha whispered as she entered the office. "It's damn good to be me."

Dr. Thompkins preferred this late afternoon "twilight hour" to catch up on paperwork and reports. With the rest of the regular nine-to-fivers gone, he was able, in his solitude, to focus without the intrusive interruptions which would derail his train of thought. He craved the silence. All of his cylinders were on full throttle when left alone with only his thoughts and his pipe. And since he'd gotten behind in his journal reviews and chart audits, he needed this time more than ever. He had gotten behind on his work due to the recent visit to the panelists and, most notably, Theodore Butler. As he had promised, he called the inept shift supervisor each week to check in on his progress and hadn't gotten a sense that he had a clue as to what the real gravity of the situation was in his vantage point of the world.

"Oh, yes sir, yes sir. Things are just swell over here, sir. Couldn't ask for a better team, that's for sure."

Dr. Thompkins would quiz Theo on the morale of the group, getting canned responses in return.

"Like a well-oiled machine, Doctor. I mean, they are really just a great, great group."

Having heard the groveling of residents and interns throughout his professional career, Dr. Thompkins was well versed in the pandering of those who were ill-prepared and in over their heads. With faux bravado, Theodore was no different, trying to convince not only Dr. Thompkins but himself that everything was as it should be.

And, in reality, Dr. Thompkins didn't care enough to delve any deeper. As long as this group was staying off of the radar, then he was satisfied with their progress. And an even better barometer of success was the absence of surprise phone calls from Samantha for several days. He felt relaxed and somewhat assured that any issues the panelists previously had must have organically worked themselves out. No news was good news as far as he was concerned. He puffed on his cutty, unfurling smoke rings above his head, as he dove into the work piled before him.

The audible *thud* outside of the office jarred him, making him jump. His pipe fell, getting ashes and unburnt tobacco on his pants and the carpet underneath his desk chair. He made no attempt to brush off the pipe's contents, as he immediately recognized the sound. What would the message be this time?

Apprehensive, he rose to his feet and made his way through the maze of papers and reports to the door. He held his hand on the doorknob, deliberating on whether to open the door hastily to potentially scare off an intruder, or slowly, so as to perhaps sneak up on whoever it was. He listened to the door before turning the knob, hoping to not hear anyone on the other side. Once the door was cracked, he was relieved not to see anyone. As expected, another brown, paper-wrapped package lay on the floor. Not bothering to try to follow whoever had left it, he picked it up and closed the office door, locking it behind him for some semblance of security.

After placing the package on top of the papers and files on his desk, he took a seat and leaned back. Recalling the contents of the last mystery package, which highlighted the obituary of his former colleague, he wondered if this was going to be a repeat message. With trembling hands, he gingerly opened the brown paper wrapping and found a newspaper with a Post-it note affixed to it. He read the words with a mixture of dread and unabashed curiosity.

Obits
(This is your last warning)

After picking up the newspaper, he went straight to the section containing the obituaries. Hastily reading the names, he froze when he saw it. He dropped the paper back onto his desk and stared at the ceiling in an attempt to grasp some sense of understanding to this confusing and disturbing message. His breath came in rapid puffs, and he rubbed his eyes before picking up the newspaper to read the obituary more closely. It took a few times of rereading to fully comprehend what he was seeing.

After all, it wasn't every day you got to read your own obituary.

Eugenia Stephenson pulled her pea-green Caprice Classic onto the on-ramp in a hurry to get home. At eighty-one years old, her family had asked—no, begged!—her to stop driving. "Ma! You've got, what did the doctor say you got? You got the macular degeneration! You shouldn't be driving. I'll drive you wherever you want to go. Ma!"

Her stubbornness had gotten her this far in life, and no one was going to tell her what she could and couldn't do. Having been a widow for the past twenty-seven years (Leroy Stephenson was just as stubborn as Eugenia, even though their family asked—no, begged!—him to stop smoking), she did things her way and there was no budging her. Doctors were pill-pushers, always "practicing" medicine, never perfecting it. She could see well enough and it wasn't like she was driving long distances. Grocery store, the rec center for bridge tourneys each Tuesday, and church.

"Hell, I could drive to those places with my eyes closed!" She prided herself in her driving skills and had never gotten so much as a warning ticket in all her sixty-five years of driving.

"No one tells Eugenia she can't drive. Harrumph!"

With a light drizzle falling, Eugenia had to squint to even see the taillights in front of her. Turning on her frayed windshield wipers, she regretted her refusal of her perceived upcharge by the oil-change mechanic only last week to replace her air filter ("That's a known scam!") and replace her windshield wipers ("Bunch of rip-off con artists. Imagine trying to do that to an old lady!").

As the shorn wipers smeared the rain across the windshield, Eugenia's thoughts about the universal thievery of car mechanics were replaced by her more recently renewed, decades-old resentment of Tricia Webster. She had yet to prove it, but it was well known to most of those in her bridge group that Tricia cheated at cards. No one wins *that* much, that consistently. That's science, not opinion. Eugenia just *knew* her nemesis was either stacking the deck, adding up points in her own favor, or somehow using sleight of hand to deal herself a winning outcome each time. It was infuriating, and Eugenia could not stand playing with her. She had contemplated quitting her bridge group so many times, but each time she thought about it, she would talk herself back in. "Why should I give that no-good bimbo the satisfaction?"

Her bad mood from losing to Tricia (again) mixed with the increasing rain made Eugenia's mood go quickly from bad to worse. Honking at the inept drivers sharing the road with her, she bobbed and weaved her Chevy from lane to lane, splashing water on the slower cars that dared to get in her way.

"Move it, slow poke!" Eugenia yelled at the traffic jammers. As the rain pelted her windshield, her vocalizations escalated, and her lack of patience (including anger at Tricia's wicked ways) grew and grew.

"Where'd you get your license? K-Mart?"

"Stay home next time, grandpa!"

"MOOOOOOOOVE!"

With each tirade, her breath steamed up the windshield.

Coupled with the incessant precipitation, faulty wipers, and blurred vision, her ability to see anything diminished to almost zero.

In fact, not until she was mere inches from the car in front of her did she finally see the brake lights and pressed both feet on the brakes. Now, Eugenia's thriftiness was legendary in the local auto maintenance circles and her bald tires and practically non-existent brake pads did little to help her in her moment of need to come to a full stop.

The police report said witnesses estimated Eugenia was going sixty-five miles per hour (it was actually closer to 70 mph) and that she did not stop as she slammed into the Dodge Ram Pickup Truck in front of her. Eugenia's Caprice absorbed the majority of the body damage, as well as, well, Eugenia herself.

As the Jaws of Life cut through the frame of the Caprice Classic to extricate Eugenia from the wreckage, she went in and out of consciousness, drifting in a peaceful dream-state, not understanding anything that was yelled at her by eager-to-help bystanders, police, fire fighters, or paramedics.

"Can you hear me?"

"Nod if you are in pain!"

"Wiggle your fingers or toes!"

"Hang in there, old timer!"

Eugenia heard none of the shouts of encouragement or directions. Instead, she blissfully floated above it all as her body was eventually lifted out of the crumpled shell of an automobile and placed on a stretcher by the EMTs. The soft rain was a comfort to her, and she gently lapped the blood tinged water as it rolled off of her face onto her lips. Once

freed from the wreckage, her body suddenly recoiled in realizing the agony it was in, and Eugenia let forth a series of
expletives and cursing that stopped everyone in their tracks.
Surely these words were not coming from this diminutive
elderly lady, were they? They were. In fact, the only thing that
was in competition with the cringeworthy volume of Eugenia's vocalizations was the graphic nature of the profanity
spewing from her bloodied mouth, which had several teeth
missing. She felt each jostle and bump of the stretcher and
expressed her dissatisfaction with the skillset of the EMTs
in a clear, unambiguous manner.

"Are you TRYING to kill me?"

"You're doing that on PURPOSE!"

"Where'd you get your EMT license, K-MART?"

As Terrell and Carlos loaded Eugenia into the back of
the ambulance, they splinted her fractured legs, put pressure on the bandage wrapped around her head to help stop
the bleeding, and gave her a healthy dose of morphine to
ease her pain. Starting fluids, they awaited direction from
D-MACS as to where to take her for treatment.

"Fifty dollars says it ain't the closest hospital."

Exiting the elevator, Dr. Thompkins looked as if he had
seen a ghost and it was still chasing him. He sped through the
winding maze of cubicles, straight toward Theodore Butler's
office. Evan and Peg both watched as he moved across the
department, his wild hair even more unkempt, face pale and
worried, coupled with a stern look of intention and determination. It was obvious he was not wanting to stop for a

casual conversation with any of the panelists as he headed to the back of the offices. Evan threw Peg an expression of concern and worry, which Peg returned. No way of knowing what had driven the medical director back to their floor, bee-lining toward Theodore Butler's office. Several other panel-ists stood as well, watching the activity with confusion and their own opinions. Murray offered up the first shot.

"That old man better slow down or he's gonna fall and break a hip."

"You think maybe this time Theo's goose is cooked?"

"I bet he's gonna fire Theo's ass."

"You keep goin', Doc! Take Murray out with him!"

Murray scowled in the direction of the last comment, but eventually he sat back down in a huff. Evan sat back down at his desk as well.

"What do *you* think that's about, nimwit? You seem to be all chummy lately with Theo and everybody. You must know. C'mon, what's happening?"

Evan slowly shook his head and turned toward Murray. "No clue. No clue at all."

"C'mon, man. You think I'm dumb? I've been watching you. All smiles to your little posse. I don't know what you are up to, but ol' Murr is gonna find out. You wait and see."

Evan stared at Murray and did his best to de-escalate his co-worker's suspicions.

"Oh ... *that*! You are just too smart, Murray. You know that? Here I was thinking I was being conspicuous and covert and there you go ... blowing my cover. I guess I might as well spill the beans ... I mean, you're going to find out anyway, aren't you?"

Murray excitedly rolled his desk chair closer to Evan, rubbing his hands in anticipation of something juicy.

Evan leaned forward. "Can you keep a secret?"

"Hey ... who do you think you're talking to here? It's me. The Murr-Man." He thumped his hand to his chest. "Think of me as your priest, your attorney, and your therapist all rolled up into one fun-lovin' guy. Spill the beans, knuckle-head."

"Well, if you must know ... It's Theo's birthday next month and several of us were thinking that it's been so stressful around here lately, what if we all chipped in and got him one of those massaging chairs for his office. We weren't sure if you'd let him know or not, so we opted to keep you out of the loop. Sorry, Murray. But now you know."

The excitement on Murray's face quickly evaporated, and he stared at Evan in disappointment and disdain. "Nah. I was right the first time I met you. You're a complete moron. Hey, do me a favor, will ya? Just continue to 'keep me out of the loop' of anything you and your gaggle of like-minded nitwits come up with, OK?"

"Sure, Murr. No problem."

Murray quickly rolled his office chair back to his desk, shaking his head and mumbling to himself. "What a Putz. What a genuine, card-carrying, no-good Putz."

Evan let out a quiet sigh of relief to have gotten Murray out of the picture. Now he could focus his attention on the new development at hand.

What was Dr. Thompkins here for, and why was he in such a hurry to meet with Theo?

He got his answer soon enough.

"Show me the detailed CFR Theodore. Now!" Dr. Thompkins addressed him with newfound sternness and command. It was amazing what seeing your name in the obituary section could do to your usual style of patience and calmness. He was seething.

"Um, the 'detailed CFR' ... the 'detailed CFR' ... oh, yeah. I got that, um somewhere. Let me see if I can sort through this to find it for you."

"You have no idea what I'm talking about, do you Theodore? Do you?" The bumbling stumblings of Theo did little to mollify his ire.

Theo sheepishly shook his head, his cheeks reddening.

"Oh, give me that." Dr. Thompkins grabbed the computer mouse and clicked a few tabs to pull up the report he wanted. "Log in. NOW!"

Theo quickly entered his log-in information and then relinquished the controls of the computer back to Dr. Thompkins. Quickly toggling through various names, he scrolled down to the most-recent patient case tabbed by the panelists.

"This one. Look."

As the screen came to life, Dr. Thompkins began his assessment of Eugenia Stephenson, assuming (correctly) young Theodore was in over his head.

"OK. What have we got here? Eighty-one-year-old white female. MVA. History of atrial fibrillation, has been on Coumadin for, let's see, aha, the past seventeen years. Also has a history of macular degeneration, osteoporosis, and hypertension. Possible early stages of dementia. OK. OK. What about the MVA ... what was logged on that?"

Once the hyperlink was clicked on, the EMTs first responder report generated onto the screen.

"Bilateral femoral fractures. Head injury. Blown right pupil. Holy crap, Theodore. What on earth?"

Theo stared blankly at Dr. Thompkins, not sure of the appropriate response.

"Um ... that sounds bad, right?" Theo fidgeted with the stapler on the desk.

Dr. Thompkins swiveled to him. "Good God, man. Are you kidding me? This old lady has a head bleed as a result of her car accident and being on long-term anticoagulants. Assuming she survives the trip to a hospital, she would either be rightly denied surgery by any neurosurgeon with half a brain or, God forbid, some rogue surgeon attempted surgery, she would languish in an ICU until eventual removal of life-sustaining therapies. But you, you, and your vagabond group of bleeding hearts score her a, what, a THIRTY-THREE?!?! Are you kidding me?"

Pulling up the detailed consolidated feedback response, the bell curve displayed on the monitor. It was decidedly a misshapen bell curve.

"So, you got one or two over here scoring, appropriately, a sixty-eight and a seventy-one as is appropriate. But who are these in this grouping? You've got some rogue reverse vigilantes in your midst, Theodore. Don't you see what is happening?"

Theo set down the stapler. His blank stare was all the answer Dr. Thompkins needed.

Pointing his finger at the grouping of low scores on the graph, he wildly circled them while addressing Theo.

"This group here, of what? Four, five, six ... six panelists were enough to skew the average and send this obvious
denial of care straight to the OR! Can't you see that? How
long has this been going on, Theodore? Can you at least tell
me that?"

His blank stare overlaid with serious processing over-
load almost resulted in black smoke coming from his ears.

"Let me see the monthly CFR numbers, Theodore. The
monthlies."

Theodore had those reports accessible more readily,
as he printed them off at the beginning of each month and
placed them neatly in a three-ring binder without looking at
them or doing any reviewing of the data whatsoever. After
pulling the binder off his shelf, he turned the page to the
most recent month and was mortified to see the numbers.

Dr. Thompkins peered closer at the page and the
dates corresponding to the dramatic drop in average
scores. "Here, right here. Same curve. Same damn curve,
you see that? This is not a coincidence, Theodore. This
is treasonous. And I'm not going down with this ship.
No, sir. Get this fixed today ... pronto. I mean NOW!"
Dr. Thompkins held his face inches from Theo's, and he
could feel is veins throbbing in his neck and forehead. He
needed to calm down if he didn't want the obit to come
true—no good actually exploding right there in the shift
supervisor's office.

Theo immediately stood at attention. "Of course, sir, of
course. I was just thinking the same thing ... the same thing.
Unbelievable. I'm on this. You can count on me. But, um, sir,
one question."

Dr. Thompkins stared at Theo, impatience and disdain coursing through his veins. "What? What is it?"

"Well, um, sir ... a few weeks back you, um, you asked me to get morale up and what not and, well, I kinda did that. And, well sir, I do feel that the morale here has just been swell, just super, sir, and, well, the date on the graph you just saw—that was the same day things started improving here. So, sir, I guess my question is this. Do you think the two go hand in hand?"

Dr. Thompkins closed his mouth and considered this a moment. Another scan of the monthly CFR and he realized young Theodore was on to something.

"Well yes, son, it appears you just might be right about that. So, let's play this out. You are tasked with improving morale that we assumed was dissension in the ranks related to Status Quotient. Then you say the morale made an uptick the same time these CFR averages plummeted? Well done, Theodore. Well done! Don't you see? This confirms it. The group of rebels took their angst out more covertly and uniformly than I gave them credit for. This was a coordinated subversion against D-MACS. Against you. And against me! End it. Now, Theodore."

At that, Dr. Thompkins quickly exited Theo's office and made a beeline toward the bank of elevators. He made no attempts to engage in eye contact or conversation with anyone on the floor. Rather, he wanted the message to be conveyed loud and clear to the entire group of panelists: Dr. Thompkins was not a fool and was not to be trifled with. He wanted every panelist who watched him march by to have a sense of intimidation and fear. And perhaps his bravado would tacitly convince the naive Quixotes, whomever they were, to end their crusade against these futile healthcare windmills and fall back in line.

After all, young Theodore was going to need all the help he could get.

Dr. Thompkins wasted no time and hurried out of the office building and on to the busy street. He raised the collar on his coat against the cold and began walking intently back toward his own office. Across the street, a driver raised his opened tinted window. He caught just a glimpse of the driver's face before it closed completely and the car sped off. A chill ran through him—he had a sense that he knew this person and was being watched.

"I'm just being paranoid," he told himself as he thrust both hands in his pockets and made quick strides down the sidewalk to his building, keeping his head down and not making eye contact with any passersby. As he walked, he glanced at the cars on the streets as covertly as he knew how. "That face looked so familiar, didn't it?" He racked his brain, trying to connect the dots. "What to do? What to do?"

As he drew closer to his building, he thought he saw the same make and model of car parked illegally across the street. Was it running? He strained his eyes, looking for exhaust fumes from the muffler on this cold day. Not seeing any, he second-guessed his paranoia and decided he was just seeing things. But ... that car. He hadn't seen a red 1980s Mercedes-Benz 380 SL convertible in quite a while and ... who in the world did he know that drove one of those? As much as he tried, he could not get the synapses to fire in sync, and he was left feeling that he knew something that he could not pull to his frontal lobe. Resigning himself to this, he knew if he stopped focusing on it, the memory would appear, and the mystery would be solved.

As he rode the elevator to his floor, he did his best to stop thinking about the familiar car and, instead, focus on the next steps to reinstate his standings with the powers that be into good graces. After exiting the elevator, he hastened to his office door, unlocked it, and closed the door behind him as fast as he could. Once he locked the door, a wave of relief and safety washed over him … until he saw the silhouette of a figure standing in his office near his desk. All at once, he realized where he had seen the red convertible before.

"Hello, Harold. I think we need to talk."

TRUTH, LIES, AND SOMEWHERE IN-BETWEEN

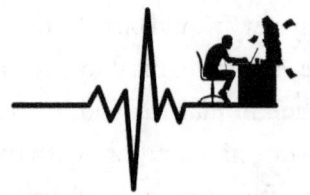

CHAPTER THIRTEEN

Evan needed to think. And for Evan, there was only one place he could go for the type of non-distracted thinking he required here and now. This kind of contemplation couldn't be done at Houlihan's Hideaway. Besides, Harry would try to problem solve for him, and Evan wasn't ready for that type of collaboration at this point. Yet having a fellow traveler who was in the thick of it with him might just be the ticket.

"Hey, Peg," he said, finding her easily, as she was sitting at her desk. Wanna go somewhere with me?"

Peg's face lit up, which made his chest feel a little funny. He rubbed at it as Peg suddenly got invested in her computer work.

He waited as she keyed a few things in, and when she stopped, she blinked up at him, her lips curving into a smile. She then casually said, "Sure, I guess."

Evan tried to hide his excitement. He'd never brought anyone there, and thinking of having Peg go with him was amazing.

With his best composed tone, he returned her blinks and then let out a sigh before responding, "Cool. Cool. Grab your coat. It's only about five or six blocks from here. We'll walk."

"Sure, yeah, OK. I'll meet you at the elevator. Or whatever."

"Yeah, that's cool. I mean, sure. Yeah … Let me grab my coat, and I'll just meet you, um, over there." Evan pointed his thumb towards the bank of elevators.

As Peg shut down her computer and walked away, Evan paused so as to not appear too hurried, then went to close up his computer station.

Murray met him there, leaning against Evan's desk, arms folded. "Good God, Evan. Was that your attempt to be Rico Suave or something? I mean, that was painful."

"Shut up, Murr. We're just going out for a bit on break. Nothing more."

"Well, based on what I just witnessed, you hit the nail on the head with that one. 'Nothing more' is about all that's going to come out of your yawn fest."

"Just co-workers, remember, Murr? Colleagues. Nothing more is *supposed* to come out of it."

"Well, I don't normally do this. But I can't stand to see such an embarrassing spectacle, even coming from you. So, if you would like, I could give you a few pointers on … you know. *You* know." To emphasize whatever it was that Evan didn't know, Murray elbowed Evan a few times in the arm.

"Thanks, Murray. I'm good though. Really. If I ever find myself in need of advice of the Casanova type, I know who to call. But this is on the level. Just co-workers."

"You really are an idiot, you know that? Knock-out like our girl Peg there and you want to stay in the friend zone. Whatever, dude. Whatever."

Evan smiled at Murray and put on his coat. "Well, I guess I'm just not as smooth as you when it comes to the opposite sex, huh?"

"Truer words have never been spoken. If Theo comes by, whadya want me to say?"

"Oh, I don't know. You're smart. You'll think of something. Maybe say, I don't know, that we went on our freaking break? Which is exactly what we are doing!" Evan tried to keep his frustration down but it was always difficult with Murray.

"Chill out, man. I'm just trying to help you out here. I won't let Theo know anything is going on between the two of you."

Evan stared blankly at Murray, doing his best to not show his increasing impatience. "Yeah, thanks Murr."

As he walked away, he heard Murray giving an unsolicited, unwelcomed, repeat performance of his pantomiming make-out session, complete with audible kisses and moans. Then came, "Oh, Peg!" and "Oh, Evan, you animal!" as Evan approached Peg at the elevators.

"He's a loser, Evan. Just ignore him." Peg gave Murray an icy stare, making him pause for only a moment, before resuming his heavy necking routine.

They both got onto the elevator and Evan punched the first-floor button.

She continued as the elevator began its descent. "Besides, we got a lot to talk about. What was all that with

Dr. Thompkins, you think?" Peg tilted her head, eyes narrowing. "I've never seen anyone so frightened yet angry at the same time. You got any idea?"

"That's what I want to go over with you. But let's get out of here first, OK?"

As they exited the building, Evan led the way, heading east at a brisk pace, thoughts swirling.

"Hey, Evan! Slow down a bit. You got me running here!"

Evan, realizing he'd been lost in his head, immediately eased up his speed.

"Oh, sorry." He came to a complete stop in the middle of the sidewalk and turned to Peg. He took a deep breath and considered her for a moment. "I'm sorry, also, for bringing you into all this. You literally just started here and now you are knee deep in this ... this ... I don't know what it is. Maybe I'm crazy."

Peg smiled at Evan and grabbed his hands, while irate pedestrians merged around them.

"It's fine. It's more than fine, Evan. Do you know this is the first time in my entire adult life that I have actually looked forward to going to work? And do you know why?"

Evan shook his head.

"Because of you. You inspire me. You have a huge heart. You are ... well, you are brave!"

Laughing, Evan began walking again at a much slower pace. Peg walked beside him, still holding on to one of his hands.

"Brave." He snorted. "That's a good one, Peg. I can't sleep over all of this—I have no idea what is happening from one moment to the next. I might even get us fired or, worse, arrested for some type of health care fraud or something, and you think I'm brave?"

Peg squeezed his hand.

"Yes, I do. All that, and more. And I'm not the only one who thinks this. Everyone who is behind you with our scoring plan, which YOU developed, feels the same. I'm behind you one hundred percent. WE are behind you one hundred percent. This is a good thing—it really is."

Relaxing, Evan realized how important Peg was in this initiative he was attempting. They continued walking, with the sun at their backs, down the sidewalk. Watching the ground as he went, he smiled at the shadows they made with their hands intertwined.

And he liked that. A lot.

"Oh! We're here." Evan pulled up short.

Peg eyed the building they were next to. "The Modern Museum of Art? I didn't know you liked art, Evan."

"I don't. Come on."

As they walked up the steps, Evan imagined they looked like a couple to anyone glancing their way. He bought two tickets, and they made their way through the crowd until he maneuvered the two of them into a room with only a few patrons.

Peg spun a slow circle. "I've never seen this work before. It's … interesting."

"I like to come here to think. No one ever really interrupts you when you're staring at something hanging on the wall."

They stood together, hand in hand, looking at squiggles in oils and charcoal as if they were deeply engrossed in the art.

Peg giggled, then let out a raucous laugh before saying loudly, "I think this one is a naked lady riding on the back of an elephant! Is this *Lady Godiva on Safari*?"

"Shhhhhhhh!" a passerby said as she scowled at them and left the room.

Peg quietly said, "Sorry" to where the shusher had been, and then smiled at Evan.

"I hoped that would give us the room to ourselves. So. What's on your mind, Evan?"

Evan smiled at Peg. He had made a wise decision in inviting Peg along with him.

"Well ... I think we're screwed."

The man standing in Dr. Thompkins' office stepped out of the shadows and into the light so that he could be seen.

Dr. Thompkins didn't know what to say.

"I know, I know. I'm supposed to be dead." Dr. Simon Corneal smiled.

"I ... I ... what in the world? I don't understand. Simon? I'm so ... so ... relieved! And confused."

Having no idea what to do in such a situation, Dr. Thompkins quickly went over and embraced him. "You're dead. And, apparently, so am I."

"Well, what did Mark Twain say? 'The report of my death was an exaggeration.' I can't believe they got to you as well. And how insulting to say I drowned in the pool at the 'Y'! How dare they! Could you think of a more offensive affront to my legacy? Bastards."

"Dammit! This is wild. I couldn't recall—at first—why the car looked familiar! I can't believe I forgot your affinity for old German clunkers. I'm so glad you're OK. But ... I just don't understand. Why ... I mean ... how—how in the world are we appearing in the obits when we are obviously very much alive and well? And what does it *mean*? Like, what is the point of it?"

"I've given a lot of thought to it, you know, since I'm dead and all, and I have a theory."

Dr. Thompkins sat at his desk and grabbed his pipe and initiated his ritual of packing tobacco and lighting it.

"Please, continue."

"Well, do you remember what I said to you at the presentation you gave about the Status Quotient?"

"Of course, Simon. I have thought about it constantly. 'Be careful—they are watching' or something of that nature. The way you had become so demonstrative of your disdain for D-MACS lately, I really just chalked it up to you having some type of breakdown or something."

"Is that what you think now?"

"Well, I don't really know what to think to be honest with you." Dr. Thompkins blew a perfect smoke ring above his head and smiled at Simon, relieved that he was OK. His smile quickly faded, however, as the gravity of the situation at hand began to weigh upon him. "So ... what is your theory?"

"First, you got anything to drink in this mess of an office?" He eyed the stacks on stacks of reports, files, and newspapers, amusement apparent on his face.

"Let's see, I've got something somewhere ..." Dr. Thompkins opened various drawers and cabinets in his office. "Here we are!"

After pulling out a bottle of scotch, he found two fairly clean glasses in another cabinet. With a healthy amount pour, he handed Simon a glass.

Holding it aloft, Simon said, "Here's to death. It's awfully overrated!"

Dr. Thompkins laughed then took a swig from his glass. He couldn't stop his grimace. "Damn, I don't know why I keep this stuff around."

"Well, it comes in handy in times like these, don't it?" Simon drained his glass and indicated he was ready for another.

Dr. Thompkins gave him another pour, then settled back into his desk chair.

"Well? Your theory?"

Simon took another sip from his glass, then sat down in the chair nearest Dr. Thompkins's desk. He swirled the contents of his glass, staring at the amber liquid for a moment before answering.

"I think we're screwed."

Aaron Gray always knew he would be around rock music in some capacity. Unfortunately, Aaron's parents had little interest in encouraging his passion, and he never got around to learning guitar or keyboard or anything. But he loved the rock scene regardless. After graduating high school (barely), he set out on the glamorous life of being a roadie. Well, *glamorous* was what Aaron had always imagined. He was surprised on multiple levels as to his career choice. First of all, he was supposed to have little interaction with the talent, as the road manager called the members of Tattooed Thunder.

"Do not look at them. Do not talk to them. And under NO circumstances do you even breathe the same air as them, you got it?"

Second of all, he wasn't supposed to fraternize with the groupies hanging around backstage, waiting for a stolen moment with the band. The road manager was explicitly clear on that as well.

"Do not look at them. Do not talk to them ..."

And third of all, the work was hard. Really hard. Electric amps, the kind of amps that generated the wattage needed to deafen any unsuspecting teenager within fifty yards of the damn things, weighed, like, a ton. And Aaron was expected to hoist them, roll them, stack them, you name it.

Yeah, it was not what Aaron had expected. On some level, though, he felt a distant connection to the band. And he did manage to snag a girlfriend or two through the years based on the mistaken expectation that a relationship with him would lead to a relationship with someone in Tattooed Thunder. Maybe not the lead singer, duh. But possibly the bass player? Once the truth was realized, Aaron would be left alone again. Which was for the best anyway, as he wasn't interested in any long-term commitment at this stage of his life.

After fifteen years as a roadie, he had paid the price with his body. Smoking (legal and otherwise) had weathered his face and aged his lungs. Drinking beer was expected of the crew, and he was known to swig with the best of them. He could pass for sixty-three rather than his actual thirty-three, especially since he had grayed in his late twenties, his long beard something of a spectacle. His stout frame (some said stout; some said obese) was heavily tattooed and devoid of any structured exercise routine. Could he lift an amp over his head? Damn straight he could. But that was the extent of his endeavors. He was rapidly heading down a dangerous road.

After each show, he and the other members of the crew would break down the set, load up the trucks, then bus it to the next show. After years on the road, his fairly sedentary lifestyle was catching up with him. Often, his legs became swollen, with occasional associated pain, but he was able to ignore it most of the time. No one had the time to hear about leg pain, nor did anyone really care. Aaron was a prisoner of his own doing. He knew no other life and didn't think any other options were available. While he had successfully convinced himself he was an invaluable member of the Tattooed Thunder family, no one else thought about him at all. It was during the set breakdown after the most recent concert that got Aaron. While lifting the lead guitarist's amp over his head, he felt a pain like he had never felt before searing across his chest. He could not catch his breath. Aaron and the amp, toppled onto the stage. Several roadies tended to Aaron, not knowing what to do.

"Did the amp land on his head?"

"Is he even breathing?"

"Why is he turning blue?"

"He's gonna pay for that busted amp, you know?"

Once the EMTs wound their way with a stretcher to the concert stage where Aaron was laying, several onlookers were watching helplessly.

"Dispatch, this is Shaver, over."

"Whatya got, Shaver?"

"Thirty-three-year-old white male. Morbidly obese. Looks like a PE. He's not breathing—currently doing CPR and about to intubate, over."

"Hold on, Shaver. What's his name, over."

"License says Aaron Gray. Sending over his info now."

"Got him. Thanks. Go ahead and tube him, and we will let you know where to head."

"Cool. He's pinking up now. Just let me know. We'll go ahead and load him and await your call"

Terrell and Carlos worked on taping the endotracheal tube over Aaron's gray beard and got him loaded onto the stretcher. It took the assistance of two other roadies, Huck and Spider, to get the stretcher off the stage and on a path to the ambulance. Aaron was, as they said, a big ol' boy.

Carlos lifted his chin at Terrell as they made their way to the truck. "Your turn, man. What you say?"

"Man, I don't even know anymore. This guy? I'll say twenty we got no lights, no siren. And three hospitals away. Easy."

Carlos studied the protruding abdomen as he bagged oxygen into the airway tube and considered the beer stains on the concert T-shirt doing little to cover the roadie's stomach.

"Yeah, man. You're right about this one. This is gonna be a 'take your time' situation. Speaking of which, you hungry?"

"Yeah, I am. Let's get him loaded, then hit up the burger joint around the corner. I heard they got a secret sauce on their smash burgers that is second to none."

"You're on."

When dispatch summoned Terrell, he responded, saying, "This is Shaver. What we doing here?"

"Hey, Shaver. Take your time. Head to Valley Community Hospital. You know where that is?"

"Yeah ... but it's been a while. Lights? Siren?"

"Negative, Shaver. Have a great night. And, oh yeah, you gotta stop by 'Smash N' Dash' around the corner from you. Have you heard about them? Got a great secret sauce, over."

"Oh, yeah. We are already on our way."

As they closed the doors on Aaron after loading him into the back of the ambulance, they made their way to the outskirts of town to the farthest hospital away from them but still in their jurisdiction.

And the secret sauce was to die for. Literally.

ROCK AND ROLL ALL NIGHT

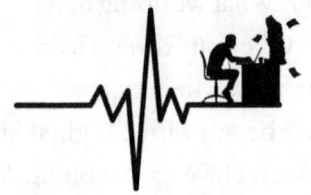

CHAPTER FOURTEEN

Theo had his computer screen on and was nervously watching the monitor. After Dr. Thompkins' tirade, he knew he had to figure out what was going on and who was causing the disruption. A new call had come in, and Theo chewed his fingernails as he awaited the tabulation. As the panelists submitted their scores, he grabbed his computer mouse and pulled up the chart.

"Let's see. Thirty-three-year-old. Pulmonary embolism with respiratory failure. Required intubation in the field. History of DVTs, obesity, smoking, positive for THC. Several unpaid parking tickets and a few arrests for assault and battery, mainly related to intoxication. No family. And he scored …?"

Theo clicked a few more screens and pulled up the CFR and …

"Whew!" Theo let out a sigh and sat back in his chair.

"The panelists got this one right. Looks like only a few tried to score him lower, but they were outliers." Theo stared at the screen and did his best to connect the dots.

Deciding he should do a head count to try and figure this out, he got up from his office chair. As he made his way around the floor, he tried his best to appear casual, seeing which panelists were here to get this one right. And which panelists were *not* here, thereby potentially sending the scores the wrong direction.

He noticed a few empty cubicles. Seeing Murray, he reluctantly stopped.

"Hey, Murr. What's shaking?"

Murray looked up from his computer monitor at Theo. Though at first his lips were twisted into a scowl, his expression instantly cleared as he sat straight in his seat.

"Oh nothing. Um, *sir.* Just working hard like I normally do. Unlike, ahem, some people." Murray darted his eyes toward Evan's empty cubicle.

Theo followed Murray's gaze and saw that not only was Evan's station empty, but also his computer monitor was off.

"Hey, where's Evan?" Theo peered over the top of the cubicle stations, trying to see if Evan was anywhere around.

Murray motioned for Theo to lean in closer.

Now normally, Theo had enough sense to not get too close to Murray's offensive aftershave and propensity for Slim Jim's. But his curiosity got the best of him. He leaned in. "Yeah?"

"Well, you didn't hear it from me. But our boy Evan here is, well, not here. As you can see. And neither is Peg." Murray wiggled his eyebrows up and down to let Theo know that the two of them were up to no good.

Theo stood and looked over the cubicles at Peg's station. Her chair was also empty and her computer monitor dark.

"Did he say where they were going?"

"No. Just that they were going on 'break.' And I think you know what that means."

Theo didn't know what that meant. He shook his head.

Murray sighed. He wrapped his arms around himself and performed a one-man make-out session, complete with arm caresses and "Oh, Evans" and "Oh, Pegs."

Theo got the picture. He was less concerned as to the inference of interoffice romances and more concerned as to these two panelists not being a part of the most recent patient scoring. Could Evan and Peg be a part of the most recent sabotage?

"Um, yeah. Thanks, Murr." Theo walked away from Murray, trying to make sense of this realization.

"You don't even care about this? C'mon, man! At least write them up! Hello? Theo?"

Ignoring Murray's lamentations, Theo continued slowly back to his office, where he sat at his desk and pulled up the CFR again on the PE patient.

As much as he didn't want to acknowledge it, he felt confident that Evan and Peg were instrumental in the latest turn of events. He wasn't sure what to do next. Maybe it was a coincidence? Maybe it meant nothing? Or maybe it meant everything.

Sitting back in his chair, he wondered how to handle this. He had always gotten along with Evan and felt that he was one of the most dependable, well-liked panelists on his team. Surely he wouldn't turn his back on D-MACS and try to challenge the most recent mandate for scoring as a beta testing site. Would he? And what about this Peg? He didn't really know her that well. While she seemed like a nice enough panelist, he didn't know enough about her to make a conclusion about her loyalty.

The more Theo thought things through, the more he doubted his own assumptions. After all, this was one patient score. Maybe the last few weeks were an anomaly and everything was going to work out fine. Theo hated confrontation—plus he didn't have enough information yet to pin this on Evan and Peg. He decided to wait and see if the score changed with their input on future patients.

Turned out, Theo didn't have to wait very long at all.

Samantha paced her office floor as she dialed the number to Regional General's lead evaluator. Her shoes squeaked with her fast turns and clicked with each step. At last the connection went through. "What's the latest, Bill? Things getting back to normal?"

"Oh, hey Samantha. Thanks for calling. Yeah, in fact, I was just going to check in with you. I don't how you did it, but it's feeling tons better down here. Only a few in the emergency department right now, and everyone's breathing a little easier." Bill let out an audible breath as if to prove his point.

"OK, good, good. I had a feeling it would ease up. Do me a favor, would you?"

"Of course, name it."

"If things go awry, let me know ASAP, OK?"

"Yes, ma'am. I definitely will."

"I mean *immediately*, Bill. If we want things to stay

copacetic, I need to know the moment you see—well, if a patient comes in who is, well, you know ... not as we would expect. You know what I mean, right, Bill?"

"Oh, of course, of course," Bill gushed. "I understand completely."

Hanging up with the lead evaluator at Regional General, Samantha felt reassured her messages were getting heard in the direction she had hoped. This was much needed positivity in light of her most recent meeting with Earl Yarborough, which did not go as well as she had expected. Previous execs she had worked for had been so passive that she wasn't sure if they even had a pulse. She was not expecting Earl to have reviewed the data before their meeting, and he was not convinced of the forward momentum Sam had tried to sell to him. He was smarter than she gave him credit for and was taken aback by his grasp of the situation.

"What in the world is going on here?" Earl shouted, throwing the latest numbers on his desk with dramatic force. Pointing his finger at Samantha, he made it abundantly clear that he wasn't disappointed. He was mad.

"And you! You told me things were heading in the right direction, remember? Well this sure as hell doesn't look like it's heading anywhere but to Shitsville, pardon my French. Wouldn't you agree, Ms. McAllister?"

Never having been called out before, Samantha was dumbfounded, and this was in front of others on the team. She paused to summon up her confidence and take control of the situation.

"Yes, sir. I can see where you are going with this. However, I have a plan. Things are already in motion to get this taken care of immediately." Samantha stared back at Earl with all the conviction she could muster. Even though she had been mistaken in Earl's understanding of the situation, she knew that displaying resolution at this moment could make or break all she had worked for thus far. She stood tall and held eye contact with him until he blinked first.

He redirected his attention to the team. "OK, then. What are all of you nimrods doing standing around here for, then? Get back to work."

As the group filed out of Earl's office, he called for Samantha to remain behind.

Her stomach twisted. Once the rest of the financial team had left, Samantha braced for Earl's tirade.

"Sam, I trust you. I really do. Just don't try to ever fool me again. Understood? I've been doing this a long time, and I know the game. Hell, I invented the damn thing. But don't try to pull any wool over my eyes again, you hear me?"

Samantha felt the heat rise as she was scolded. She had never been spoken to like this and was unsure of how to respond. She decided to take it as a learning experience and be all the wiser for it in the future.

Plus, her next steps with Dr. Thompkins would provide satisfactory results, she was certain.

In reflecting on this moment, and hearing from Bill Wilson that her strategy was working, she garnered a renewed sense of control. Now was not the time to take the foot off of the gas. Staring out of her office window, she contemplated her next steps. They would need to be calculated and timed perfectly to hit fourth quarter numbers.

"They haven't seen nothin' yet," Sam said as she opened

up a bottle of Merlot and gave herself a healthy pour. *You got to take the little wins as they come, don't you?*

Theodore Butler had never taken the time to marry. Well, that was his justification for never actually having any prospects. "Married to my work," was Theo's standard answer whenever asked about his lack of relationship-building. "Besides, I like the freedom to go anywhere I want whenever I want." Theo never went anywhere, however, as he really only liked the freedom of sitting alone in his studio apartment in his boxers and eating frozen dinners while watching game show reruns. He could be counted on to mostly watch *Jeopardy* reruns as he had memorized most of the answers. As a *Jeopardy* purist, he only watched Alex Trebek era shows.

As Theo sat down to watch season thirty-five, episode fourteen with his piping-hot Salisbury Steak Hungry Man TV dinner, he felt as content and confident as he ever had.

"Who is Dinah Shore?"

"What is the Great Wall of China?"

"What is nitrous oxide, Alex?"

Rattling off the answers, Theo felt good. No, let's not kid ourselves here. Theo felt great.

The knock on his apartment door startled him and caused an immediate fracture of his nighttime ritual and reverie. He shuffled to the door in his boxer shorts, tattered robe, and slippers. There, he peered through the peephole to see if he recognized the intruder. No one was visible.

He opened the door and looked up and down the hall.

"Stupid Robinson kids," he muttered, assuming it was a prank knock from the surly preteen twins who lived in apartment 305. As he began to close the door, his eyes happened to see the brown paper wrapped package at his feet. He picked it up, then shuffled back inside his apartment, locking the door on his way. After tossing the package on the cluttered kitchen table, he sat back down in his recliner to finish his dinner and amaze the studio audience with his brilliant recollection of little-known trivia.

"Who is Pope Pius the ninth?"

But his heart was no longer in the show or the congealing brown-gravy-soaked formed meat. Why would he get a package? He never ordered anything online and wasn't expecting any deliveries. Sitting forward in his recliner, he looked over at the package on the kitchen table.

Theo placed his dinner back on the TV tray and went over to the package. The brown paper had no label or return address on it. Just a message handwritten in Sharpie:

Mr. Theodore Butler

Not knowing what to make of it, he decided to open it to find out the package's contents. With trepidation, he cautiously opened the wrapper to find a newspaper inside. Stuck to the newspaper was a Post-it note with only one word written with the same black Sharpie:

Obits

It had been years since Theo had seen an actual newspaper, much less read one. "Do people still read these things?" Theo asked himself as he struggled to find the section of the paper containing the obituaries. As he quickly turned each page, his curiosity grew more and more. Finally, in the section of the paper called Lifestyles (*Well, that's a funny place to put death notices, don't you think?*), Theo came to the obituaries. As he slowly read each name, he let out an exasperated sigh.

"Why would someone give me a newspaper to look at the obituaries?" Theo questioned out loud, beginning to think it was those Robinson boys again. Then he saw the name and froze, tears welling in his eyes. He immediately picked up the phone and called his sister.

"Hello? Is that you, Theo? You haven't called me in months! How are you?"

"How am I? How am I? I have to find out in the paper that Ma is dead? Why didn't you call me?"

"What on earth are you talking about? I'm sitting with her right now, you dummy."

Theo stopped his crying and paused, unable to process what was going on. "Well, I'm looking at the paper and right here, in black and white, is Ma's obituary. 'Mrs. Estelle Butler, 81, passed away in her sleep surrounded by her loved ones ... 'Survivors include Theodore Butler (son), Francine Morrison (daughter) and son-in-law Samuel Morrison' ... and so on."

"Must be some other Estelle Butler who passed away. Hold on ... Ma! Ma! Here, take the phone. It's Theo. THEO! Your son? Good grief, here, Ma."

"Hello? Hello?"

Hearing his mother's voice, Theodore began crying all over again, relieved to hear her and silently vowing to stay in closer contact with his mother and sister from this moment on. As she rambled on about her lumbago and his sister's terrible cooking, he silently recanted his vow to stay in closer contact, remembering why he had become somewhat estranged in the first place.

"Yeah, Ma, I, um, sorry, I gotta go. Just wanted to check in on you two. Bye."

"What? Theo? Is that you? Francine! Why is he getting off the phone? What is going on? Oh, my lumbago!"

As Theo hung up, he tried to make sense of everything. Sitting back down in his recliner, he pushed his dinner away and turned off the television. *Someone sent me this newspaper as a message. I just know it. There can't be another 81-year old Estelle Butler with the same named children. How? What?* Theo sat in silence, worried about the message. Was someone threatening him? Would harm come to his mother if he didn't do something? What was going on? Staring at his half-eaten dinner, he had more questions than answers and decided that only one person in his circle of contacts would possibly be able to help shed light on the situation. Folding the newspaper back in the brown paper wrapping, he decided that another phone call was in order. He just hoped he would know what was happening and be able to tell him what to do.

Staring at the painting in front of them, Peg and Evan could have been two art students engrossed in the use of brushstrokes and unblended colors, trying to elicit the secrets contained within the framed work from over one hundred years ago.

Peg squinted at the painting to try and make out what the artist was trying to create.

"You know," Evan got her attention, "I have a theory about this type of painting."

She tilted her head, trying to see from a different angle. "Yeah? Please share. I don't know *what* to make of this."

"I think the artist had crappy paint brushes. Then he tried to pass off this painting as something that he intended to do. But in all reality, he was just cheap and got some brushes down at the local French dollar store."

Peg let out a loud laugh, eliciting another "Shhhhhhhh!" from a passerby.

"Sorry! Sorry!" Peg said as she tried to contain her laughter. She was glad Evan had the same uncultured view of high-end art that she had. She had been worried she was the only one who didn't "get" the classic piece hanging on the wall in front of them. It made her like him all the more.

She nudged him with her shoulder. "So, what do we do now?"

"I'm not sure, Peg. I think Dr. Thompkins is getting wise to our scoring system. I think we'll need to proceed with caution, don't you think? I mean, I've only seen the director a few times—and never as enraged as he was up there when he went to meet with Theo. Can't think what else it would have been about if it wasn't our scoring. Did I tell you I went to see him recently?"

Peg spun toward Evan. "You did what?"

"Yeah … shortly after he gave the presentation on Status Quotient, I went to see him at his office. He gave me a bunch of malarkey, the same stuff I gave you when you were so upset about it all."

Relief coursed through her. "I *knew* that wasn't you

talking!"

Evan's eyebrows climbed.

"Oh, my goodness. No, I mean it didn't sound like something you'd say! This makes me feel so much better. So what do we do to 'proceed with caution'? Do we go back to adding in Status Quotient and effectively killing these innocent people? I mean, just because they aren't rich or famous or anything doesn't mean they should be shunned, right?"

Evan and Peg meandered to the next set of paintings. Staring at the picture, Evan crossed his hands behind his back and then leaned in. "Is that a lady in a boat in a lake? I thought at first I liked this, but now I'm not sure what I'm looking at."

"It's so muddled, I don't know what it is!"

Pointing to the picture, Evan said, "This. This is what I feel like right now. Everything is muddled and confused. I need clarity, Peg. I need things to come into focus and I don't know … I don't know …" Trailing off, Evan ambled to the next piece of framed artwork.

Peg walked up next to him and placed her hand in his.

Evan gripped her hand and turned to her, staring at her intently.

"I don't know what to do next, Peg. But I do know that I am glad to have you to figure it out with. You are one of the smartest panelists I've ever met. Seriously."

Peg smiled. "Smarter than Murray?"

They both laughed, eliciting another "Shhhhhhhh!"— this time from a security guard.

Evan whispered to Peg, "Yes, believe it or not. Smarter than Murray. I think the fact that you are so new to this, it gives you a fresh perspective that I am afraid I've lost. I was so wrapped up in the science and the pursuit of making healthcare better in my mind that I allowed myself to be a part of the problem. Your insight and ideas could be just the ticket to figuring out how to get us out of this mess."

Peg blushed, unaccustomed to praise, especially from someone she admired. And liked.

"That means a lot, Evan. It does." Letting go of his hand, she meandered to the next masterpiece on the wall.

Evan followed. "And this, this of course, is the classic rendering of a bowl of fruit. Or (squinting) perhaps a bowl of Lucky Charms. I can't really tell."

"Shhhhhhhh!" came from another patron as Ethan and Peg both laughed.

"All I know is, between the two of us, I bet we can figure out how to change the system for good. Wait, Evan, you're so smart—don't you have access to the input tablatures that we use? You showed me some sort of matrix during orientation. I had no idea what it all meant at the time, but isn't that how the scoring is inputted? I mean, could you somehow go in, behind the scenes, and change the scoring? And not have it traced to you? Is that possible?"

Evan stopped and stared at Peg, his eyes sparkling. "I *do* have access. You're right! I could go in and change it so those of us who are 'false' scoring could give a new score that would look correct to the higher ups ... but the others, like Murray, would be scoring what they think is correct, but it would give an artificially changed score. So they seem like the saboteurs! You are brilliant, Peg!" He leaned over and gave Peg a kiss on the cheek before he knew what he was doing. Sheepishly, he pulled back. "I'm sorry, Peg. That was out of line."

Peg smiled, placing her hand on her cheek where the kiss had landed. She then leaned up and gave him a return kiss, only hers landed on his lips.

Blushing, Evan flashed her a huge grin. She'd never seen him look so happy.

The two of them, hand in hand, walked out of the gallery. In her head, Peg chanted, "Newfound confidence, a newfound plan, and a newfound love." *Can it be?*

They spoke about more details of the plan, laughing out loud at the audacity of this new twist.

"Shhhhhhhh!"

LIGHTS, CAMERA, ACTION!

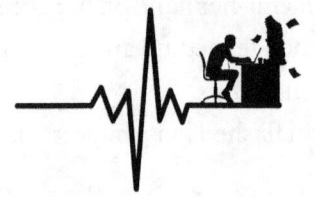

CHAPTER FIFTEEN

Hanging up the phone, Dr. Thompkins turned to Dr. Corneal. "Did you hear all of that?"

Simon nodded. "Sounds like someone else got the 'obituary' treatment?"

"Yes. That was the young man I've been working with at D-MACS—the shift supervisor—he received the same type of brown-paper-wrapped newspaper. But the obituary was not his; it was his mother's. He said he phoned her and spoke with her, so he knows it was fake. He's as confused as we are. How is this happening, Simon? I mean, what do you make of it all? Who or what is behind all of this?"

"Well, let's go over what we know definitively." Looking about the office, Simon found a flip chart on an easel in the corner underneath three tattered raincoats. After tossing the coats to the side, he flipped the pages on the chart until he found a blank sheet.

Dr. Thompkins pointed to a coffee cup on his desk that contained markers and pens.

Simon grabbed a marker, letting out a snicker when he

eyed the cup. "Seriously? 'World's Best Doctor'? You know I always got the better grades back in med school, right?"

"Grades aren't everything. Anyway, it was a gift from a grateful patient years ago. Focus, Simon, focus."

"OK, OK, OK. What do we know?"

As they spoke, he created a bulleted list on the flip chart. They began by listing the agreed upon assumptions. They continued to identify the known, objective facts as any good doctors would:

1. *Simon complains to D-MACS Medical Review Board—receives obit about self*
2. *Harold gets call from Samantha—receives same obit about Simon*
3. *Harold works with Theodore Butler—receives obit about self*
4. *Theodore Butler's scores go down—receives obit about his mom*

They stared at the flip chart, trying to find a common link.

"You complained to everyone and his brother about Status Quotient, and we all blew you off. Then you received a newspaper containing your own obituary. Obviously someone was trying to shut you up. But you spoke with many, many people, correct?"

"Right. Then you spoke with Samantha McAllister, and she told you—what did you say? 'I've done my part; now you do yours.'? What did that mean, you think?"

"She had a chance meeting with one of the panelists, I believe. A young man named Evan. She said I needed to watch out for him, calling him an 'idealistic vigilante,' I think. She expressed concern that he could possibly cause trouble with the other panelists."

"Well?" Simon tapped his closed pen against the pad. "Was she right?"

"About Evan? Oh, I don't know. I know I had a previous conversation with Samantha about my concerns regarding Evan, but I don't know. I never got a sense that he had the wherewithal to mobilize any issues among the group. However, the timing *is* right. It's possible Evan is a point person to focus our attention on."

Simon wrote "*Evan*" and underlined it on the flip chart.

"So, at the same time, you get a newspaper describing *my* death. Do you think our Samantha had anything to do with that?"

"I mean, it's possible. She was the last person I spoke with before receiving it. Still doesn't really explain number three. I mean, what on earth happened to make me of all people deserve to receive an obituary warning? I had followed up with Theodore Butler, and he gave the impression that things were improving with the panelists. I hadn't spoken with Ms. McAllister in a while. I just don't see how this is all connected. Did you ever have any dealings with her?"

Simon rubbed the stubble on his chin and closed his eyes. "Well, let's see. She is the new hire by Earl Yarborough, right? I do recall having a few conversations with her now that you mention it. Shortly after your presentation about Status Quotient if I'm not mistaken. To be honest, I didn't really know who she was. She called me a couple of times, saying it was at the behest of Earl, and told me ... what was it she told me?"

Staring at the ceiling, Simon made a humming noise in the back of his throat, then snapped his fingers. "'What's at stake!' That's what it was. She called me one night and gave me the riot act, and I didn't really pay too much attention to her. I thought she was an assistant or something of the CEO. But I do recall her saying, 'You better get on board and understand what's at stake here.' I wondered at the time who she was to tell me what to do. I was perplexed by her role and all. How about you? Have you had much interaction with this Samantha?"

Dr. Thompkins sat up straight in his chair. "Yes! Yes! She told me the same thing! When she called me about Theo, she said the exact same thing. I needed to convince Theo of 'what's at stake.' She was quite emphatic about it as well. I didn't give a lot of thought to what exactly she was referring to. She gave me the impression that the success of my latest grant was on the line, so I thought she was indirectly telling me to toe the line or I would lose some of my funding. But it's possible she was speaking in more global terms. What do you think?"

Simon shook his head slowly and pointed to the flip chart. "I don't know. I just don't know. But the answer has to be up there somewhere, don't you think?"

They sat in silence, staring at the list on the flip chart. What was the common link to it all? After a few minutes of pipe smoking from Dr Thompkins and some beard stubble scratching from Dr. Corneal, Simon finally stood.

He smiled at Dr. Thompkins and tapped on the name *"Evan"* on the page. "How well do we know this Evan? You like him? You trust him?"

Dr. Thompkins slowly shrugged. "I guess so. Like I said, he never seemed like much of a pot stirrer if you know what I mean. Self-deprecating. Company man. But benign nonetheless. Why do you ask?"

Simon took his marker and circled Evan's name several times. "I think you and I need to meet with this young man. He might be the missing link to all of this. If he's as decent as you indicate, then perhaps he shares in our distrust of where D-MACS is heading and how Status Quotient is the catalyst to it all. What do you say? Want to go pay a little visit to our boy Evan here?"

As the pipe plumes rose to the ceiling like smoke signals, Dr. Thompkins realized his colleague was right. Staring at the flip chart with Evan's name circled like a bullseye, he felt a sense of relief that Simon's perspective was spot on.

Smiling, he slid the "World's Best Doctor" coffee cup toward Simon. "Here. I think this actually does belong to you after all."

Laughing, he pushed it back towards Dr. Thompkins. "Keep it, Harold. Just figure out where we can meet up with this panelist. Any idea where he hangs out?"

"I think I have an idea. Grab your coat. We're going to a bar."

As Evan and Peg entered Houlihan's, Harry waved excitedly to the two, beckoning them to the bar.

They sat down at barstools and Harry raised his hand to shield his eyes from an imaginary sun and squinted hard. "I know I've seen this boy somewhere before, but that couldn't be my nephew with such a pretty young lady, could it?" Restraining his eyeroll, Evan grabbed his stomach and faked a large laugh. "Ha, ha, Harry. You are just too funny. Harry, this is Peg. Peg, this is my crazy uncle Harry. Harry smiled with pride and began instinctively wiping the spotless wooden bar in front of them. "It's nice to see you, Peg! What can I get you two to drink?"

Peg looked inquisitively at the various bottles and taps behind the bar. "Well, what do you recommend, my good barkeep?"

"That all depends, little lady. Are you looking to remember or to forget?"

Peg bit her lip and wrinkled her brow in deep thought. "I'm actually wanting to remember *to* forget. Got anything for that?"

"That's my specialty!" Harry winked at Evan. "I like this one, squirt!".

As Harry went to prepare it, Peg leaned to Evan. "I like your uncle. He really loves you. You can tell."

Evan smiled. "Yeah, he's a good guy. He's helped me out a lot through the years. I've always trusted his advice   he's my go to when I need to decompress or just vent."

"It's good to have someone like that you can trust. And he's so funny!"

Evan gave her the most serious look he could muster. "Peg. Please. Don't encourage him."

Harry brought over the drinks, placing a glass of sauvignon blanc in front of Peg and a vodka and tonic in front of Evan. A colorful paper umbrella stuck out of his glass.

Laughing, Peg said, "See! You're hilarious, Harry!"

Evan tried to scowl but couldn't stop the chuckle. "Nice, Harry. Real nice." He sheepishly discarded the blue and pink and green cocktail umbrella down the bar. "You're a riot."

Harry bowed to them. "I'll be here all week!" he exclaimed, then blew kisses to them and to everyone else at the bar, basking in his imagined accolades. As he made his rounds, he sang "Make 'Em Laugh" from *Singing in the Rain* loud enough for the whole bar to cover their ears.

Before long, Harry had returned to his station at the bar, polishing the wood around their drinks with his dish towel. "So, what's the latest with you both?"

Peg set her wine glass back on the bar and told Harry all about the art museum and what a "wonderful" guide Evan was. "My all-time favorite experience at a museum. Hands down!"

"Do tell, young lady. What was your favorite part? Abstract art? Watercolors? Are you a Baroque fan?"

"Well, if I have to be honest, my favorite was having all the serious, snobby art patrons hiss 'shushes' at us!"

Harry laughed with the two of them. "That's my nephew!" Patting Evan on the back of the hand, he gave out a sigh. "I was worried you were turning into an art aficionado or something. You still like to go there to think, right?"

Evan nodded. "Yep. And now Peg has joined the art guild as well. She really helped me out today, giving me some great ideas on next steps at work." He smiled at Peg and gave her hand a squeeze.

"Well, that is great news, Squirt. I'm happy for you. I'm happy for you both! Y'know what, drinks are on me tonight, how about that?"

"How about that." Evan shook his head while silently laughing. He hadn't paid for a drink at Houlihan's, well, ever. Harry always insisted.

"Oh, my goodness, thank you, Harry! That is just too kind of you!" Peg exclaimed.

Evan let Harry soak in the gratitude.

"I'll leave you two to enjoy. Oh look! Other customers are here too!" As a seasoned barkeep, Harry's timing was always impeccable—he knew when it was time to engage and when it was time to let others be. Wiping the wooden bar as he left, he threw a wink at Evan.

Raising his glass, Evan smiled at Peg. "Here's to an amazing day and our next steps to success."

Peg raised her wine glass and returned the toast. "And here's to the most amazing guy I've ever met."

Evan immediately scowled and scanned the room. "Who? Who are you talking about?" He then grinned.

"YOU!" Peg gently poked Evan and then rested her hand back on his.

Evan felt confident and at peace as he basked in the glow of being with Peg. The plan that Peg had helped develop was going to work, he just knew it. Evan had failed to mention to Harry that after the trip to the art museum, they had returned to work to finish out their day. He was able to make the changes to the input tablature that ran in the background of the panelists' worksheets. Having been given Theo's password years ago (long story that came down to Theo being lazy), Evan was able to access the password protected operations section and easily manipulate the calculations that would be used by each panelist. Those in Evan and Peg's inner circle would be able to enter reviews of the patient charts as normal. Those outside of their group would be entering scores as well, but their tablatures would now result in lower scores. Anyone looking at the panelists scores en masse would think that *they* would now be the ones who were causing the aggregate score to be lower, not Evan and Peg's ragtag team, even with Status Quotient at play. Now if anyone were to dive deeper into each panelist's calculations, his group would look innocent. It was a stroke of genius and Evan had Peg to thank for the cunning idea.

As they chatted and sipped their complimentary drinks, Evan felt content. Life was finally going his way, and he wanted to enjoy every minute of it. It wasn't until he felt the tap on his shoulder that his dreamlike state was shattered.

"Hey, Evan. We need to talk."

Joining Dr. Thompkins and another man at a table away from the bar, Evan felt as if he and Peg were being called to the principal's office. As they sat down, Evan strained to understand how their newest plan had unraveled so quickly.

Evan tried not to look guilty. *There hasn't even been a new calculation done since changing the input tablature, so how in the world could they know? Did they know? Maybe they didn't know. Maybe this is something else. Be calm, Evan, be calm.*

Facing Peg, Dr. Thompkins introduced himself. "Young lady, I do believe I have had the pleasure of meeting you before. You rescued me from that unfortunate young man. Murphy? Marley?

"Murray," Peg said.

"Ah yes, indeed. I'm Dr. Thompkins, in case it slipped your memory."

"Oh yes, I remember. I'm Peg, in case you forgot. But yes, that was on your way to meet with Theo." She cocked her head. "You just met with him again a little more recently."

Dr. Thompkins nodded without elaborating.

The other man then extended his hand to Peg, then Evan. "Allow me to introduce myself. I am Dr. Simon Corneal. I work, er, *worked* with Dr. Thompkins on the D-MACS Medical Review Board. That is, until I died most unexpectedly."

"Don't forget, Simon, I'm dead as well!"

Evan swung his gaze to Peg, who widened her eyes and shrugged. The doctors let out a quick laugh, then explained how their obituaries were delivered to them in paper parcels. They went on to explain their theories as to the packages' origins.

Dr. Thompkins leaned forward. "And this, Evan, is where you come in."

Raising his hands, Evan stammered, "I ... I didn't write any obituaries. I mean, I don't even know how one would go about creating a fake one. It wasn't me!"

"Oh, no, no, no, Evan." Dr. Thompkins shook his head. "We don't think you had anything to do with *that* per se. No, we wanted to meet with you because your name came up a few times while Simon and I were brainstorming earlier. After all, *you* are the one who came to me with your concerns about Status Quotient. And *you* had a recent chance meeting with Ms. Samantha McAllister."

Peg quirked an eyebrow at Evan. "So who is this Samantha, huh?"

Evan was baffled. "I have no idea who you are talking about. Who is Samantha McAllister?"

"She works closely with our CEO, Earl Yarborough, in the central office. We believe she might be the common link to all of this and maybe is the brains behind the operation, so to speak." Dr. Thompkins rapped his knuckles against the tabletop. "She told me she met you, actually, and had a conversation about your role at D-MACS here in this, um, 'fine' establishment. Do you recall that?"

Evan widened his eyes as he remembered the discussion Harry had facilitated not too long ago with the woman at the bar. "Yes, I did speak with a woman here at Houlihan's not too long ago. I'd been telling my uncle, the owner of this bar, about my struggle with what we were being asked to do at D-MACS. Then a lady came in, and Harry invited her to give her opinion on my concerns. I thought it was harmless—an outsider's unbiased thoughts on it. I spoke in generalized terms, of course. In fact, I don't know if she even knew where I worked. Just told her it was a 'government job,' actually."

"Oh, she most definitely knew where you worked." Dr. Thompkins gave a sharp nod. "The way she described the meeting to me, I'm sure it was just a coincidence that she ran into you. But she took full advantage of the situation to get some insight on how a panelist was feeling about their role at D-MACS and, unfortunately, how they felt about Status Quotient. I mean, no matter the 'vagueness' of the content of the conversation, I am quite sure she was able to quickly glean your role in the organization. But what I—I mean what *we*—want to know is, what did she say to *you*? Was she concerned? Angry? Anything?"

"No, not that I can recall. I mean, Harry had teed it up, so to speak, that I was struggling with a new initiative at my job so, yes, you're right that if she already knew about the introduction of Status Quotient, then she would have known what I was talking about. But, no, she wasn't upset about anything. She was polite and asked me a few questions about ... about—wait a minute!"

Both Simon and Dr. Thompkins sat more upright in the booth. Leaning in, they waited as Evan processed his thoughts.

"I thought it a little strange at the time, but, heck, I didn't pay it any mind. She asked a few questions about *you*, Dr. Thompkins."

"Me? She actually said my name to you?"

"Well, no, not by name. But she asked about how much input I got from my superiors and whether any feedback came from anyone higher up in my company. I told her I had actually spoken with my director recently about my concerns. Was that bad?"

Both Dr. Corneal and Dr. Thompkins sat back in their booth, nodding in unison.

"That's got to be it. It's just got to be. She used Evan here—sorry kid—but she used him a bit to find out about you. Don't you see? She was trying to get a sense of your commitment, Harold, don't you think?"

Dr. Thompkins wrinkled his brow. "It's possible she could have been wanting to see my level of loyalty." Turning back to Evan, he leaned in. Just then, they were interrupted by Harry.

"Hello, old timers! I'm Harry, owner of Houlihan's

Hideaway. I'm also Evan's uncle. You four look like you are trying to solve the problems of the world. Well, we got sort of a rule about seriousness around here. See the sign over the bar there?" He pointed out the hand painted sign with a caricature of a clown in a cowboy hat.

No Serious Talk in These Here Parts.
I'm Serious About That!
Seriously!

Dr. Thompkins and Dr. Corneal offered up a weak smile.

"There! That wasn't so hard, was it? As friends of Evan here, your first round is on me. What can I get you two parched partners?"

After getting their drink orders, Harry moseyed back to the bar with an exaggerated swagger.

Dr. Thompkins eyed Evan. "Your uncle is, um, something else."

"Oh, he's a good guy. He loves his job and, well, he's old school that way. Anyway, what were you going to say just then?"

"Think real hard on this one, Evan. Exactly what did you say to Samantha about *me*? This is important."

Evan reflected on it. "It was actually all good, Dr. Thompkins. I mean, you and I had recently had that conversation in your office, and I told her you and I had spoken and, well, you did your best to convince me of the importance of the newest initiative I was struggling with. That's the words I used. 'Did his best to convince me.' That's exactly what I said. I promise."

Dr. Corneal and Dr. Thompkins both stared at Evan, and he felt they were both doing a mental dissection of his character. He thought maybe he passed muster when they both gave a sharp nod.

"Well, Harold. Here's what I think. I think Samantha felt good about your commitment after speaking with Evan. After all, you didn't receive your obit until, when? Wasn't it a week or two later, after the scores started dropping?"

Evan and Peg looked at each other, then sheepishly slid down slightly on their side of the booth.

"What? What do you know about the—wait a second. It was you two, wasn't it!"

"Peg had nothing to do with this, sir. It was all my doing, I swear."

Grabbing Evan's hand, Peg interrupted. "*We* did this. We did this, us, and a few others on the floor who were concerned about this new plan to save a few bucks and not save a few lives. We had to, we just had to, you know?"

The tension was interrupted as Harry appeared and placed the two frosty mugs in front of the two doctors. "Want any cocktail peanuts or chips to go with those ice-cold delicacies?"

"Um, no thanks. This is great. Thank you."

Evan eyed Harry in a "leave us be" way.

Harry responded with a wink. "Well, if you need anything else, I'm right over there behind the bar. Ask for Harry!"

The four of them took a sip of their drinks as Harry walked away.

"Does he have an off switch or anything?" Dr. Thompkins asked incredulously to Evan.

"Not that I'm aware of. Again, he's really a great guy."

"I'm sure he is. But what were you saying? What exactly did you all end up doing that put me front and center in the obituaries?"

Evan and Peg explained to Dr. Corneal and Dr. Thompkins the scoring sabotage they initiated, as well as the most recent development of changing the input tabulation formula. The two doctors remained quiet, sipping on their beers. Then everyone leaned in, and they got down to business.

Before leaving the bar, the four of them had developed a foolproof plan.

At least they hoped it would be. They were laughing and enjoying themselves when Harry treated them each to a second round.

After all, Harry was the ultimate barkeep.

TANGLED WEB WE WEAVE

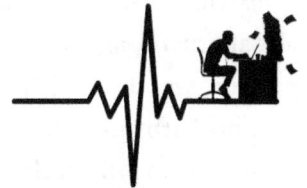

CHAPTER SIXTEEN

Jimmy stared at his calculator in disbelief. "That's malarkey. Uh-uh. No way. Over five hundred thousand? Uh-uh. Malarkey."

But the numbers, they didn't lie. On a whim, Jimmy Coltrane had decided to calculate how many cigarettes he had smoked in his lifetime. Let's see ... starting at age fourteen, probably only smoked a pack a week since he had to steal money to buy the damn things, and he figured he did that for about four years. Then, after high school, he got pretty good at smoking every day, going through about a pack a day for, oh, let's say ten years. Once he got divorced the second time, he ramped up his smokes to two packs a day. And he never looked back. Had been about thirty-five years. Really? *Time flies, I guess.* And his weathered face showed it.

Staring in the mirror at his wrinkled face and sallow complexion, Jimmy felt every bit of his sixty-two years. Plus a few. Taking in a deep breath, he triggered a coughing fit. He could count on a good five-minute "cough-a-thon" (as he called them) first thing every morning. While at first he'd felt some sense of alarm at this daily ritual, after a few years, he'd grown accustomed to it. In fact, he had gotten to where he could time the coughs with such a high degree of accuracy he knew when to take another drag off his morning smoke.

When the temperature was too cold, he preferred to host the "cough-a-thon" in his bathroom so as to have a sink to spit into. But on a nice morning like today, Jimmy could be counted on to sit on his front porch steps. He liked to feel the sun on his face while coughing and spitting onto the sidewalk. Most regular delivery workers, like the mailman, the pizza delivery boy, and the FedEx guy, had learned from experience to NOT step on the sidewalk in front of Jimmy Coltrane's house when he was outside. But, let's face it, he didn't really care.

His personal physician, Dr. Chan, had diagnosed Jimmy with chronic obstructive pulmonary disease several years ago and had pleaded with Jimmy to put down the cigarettes, to no avail. "You've got to stop smoking, Jimmy. Look! Look at those lungs on the right." He jabbed his finger at a poster from the American Lung Association hanging on the wall. "That'll be you if you keep smoking like this."

Jimmy had shrugged. "You gotta die sometime, doc. Might as well enjoy it while you can! Cough! Cough!"

Staring at his latest contribution to the phlegm on the sidewalk, Jimmy finally felt a twinge of concern. He had noticed the blood tinge for the first time a few weeks ago but dismissed it then as a flare up of bronchitis. "It's nothing but bronchitis" he'd tell anyone who would listen while smoking, hacking, and spitting.

"Beautiful morning, ain't it Jimmy? Here's your mail,"

Owen Jackson, the USPS mail carrier, said as he sidestepped Jimmy's pile of expectorant by walking in the grass next to the sidewalk. "You know, you ought to quit those things. They'll kill you one day." He handed him a few envelopes.

"You gotta die sometime ..." You know the rest.

Tossing the mail to the side, Jimmy got up to go grab another pack of Viceroys but got lightheaded and winded. Jimmy attempted to grab a hold of the banister on the porch but missed, collapsing instead. His coughing worsened and he had a hard time catching his breath.

"You OK there, Mr. Jimmy?" Owen called from his position on the street in front of Jimmy's house.

Jimmy couldn't respond.

Owen dropped his mailbag and ran to the front stoop. Unfortunately, he ran straight up the sidewalk. When his orthopedic shoes stepped in Jimmy's blood-tinged mucus, the mail carrier slipped and fell to the ground in a heap. Hitting his head on the sidewalk, Owen Jackson was knocked unconscious.

Attempting to look over at the mail carrier, Jimmy had a difficult time checking on Owen as he was unable to move closer. His wheezing and coughing seemed to have no end in sight. Jimmy was stuck on his porch, trying to troubleshoot how to help the mailman *and* himself as well. As his breathing became more and more labored, Jimmy became less and less aware of his surroundings. The hypoxia eventually caused Jimmy to black out, lying semi-prone on his porch with his back against his front door.

When Julie Ackerman, on her morning walk, passed by Jimmy's house, she just happened to notice the two prone bodies, one lying on the sidewalk and one curled on the front porch. When she screamed, several more passers-by came to see what the ruckus was about. Although the first call to 9-1-1 was, erroneously, for a double homicide, a few good Samaritans were able to revive the fallen mail carrier who had a small lump on the back of his head. A few others tended to Jimmy while awaiting an ambulance. At first, they had assumed Jimmy was already dead, due to his dusky complexion. However, upon closer inspection, he was shallowly breathing and had a faint pulse.

When Terrell and Carlos arrived on the scene, Julie told them her theory as to what had happened, letting them know that Mr. Jimmy was the one that needed the most urgent attention. "And, by the way, Terrell and Carlos, when you go up the sidewalk, best watch where you step."

Logging on to her computer, Samantha was eager to see if her hard work was, at last, paying off in a sustained way. An interminable amount of time passed before the D-MACS logo appeared on the home screen. She was anxious to determine if Theodore Butler had gotten the message. Having the highest security clearance with sign on and passcode, she quickly toggled through the various startup screens until she found the icon for viewing live scoring for new charts being generated. As her cursor blinked, she saw that a new patient review was about to be listed and tabulated. Samantha had no healthcare experience and was not interested in learning now. She only wanted to know what the final score would be and to see if it would be high enough to keep the patients from using up valuable healthcare dollars that could be spent elsewhere. Impatiently, she waited.

Logging on to the computer in his office, Dr. Thompkins was eager to see if Evan's new manipulation of the input tabulation formula would pay off without notice. Simon Corneal pulled an office chair closer to the desk in order to see as well. After what seemed like a lifetime, the "D-MACS" logo appeared on the home screen. Dr. Thompkins clicked his way through various icons and folders until he was on the screen for viewing the live scoring of a new chart. As medical directors of D-MACS, both he and Simon had enhanced access and were able to see the same information that was going to be reviewed by each panelist.

Anxious to see if this new plan worked, he grabbed a can of tobacco, which he slowly packed into his pipe. After lighting it, he puffed fresh plumes above his head. He kept an eye on the blinking icon, waiting for the next patient review to be posted. He hoped they would not have to wait long.

As Theo logged on to his desk computer, he was panicking. What would happen next to him if the panelists did not score correctly? Would he be able to determine who was manipulating the scores? As he waited for his D-MACS logo to appear, he decided to walk through the floor to see which panelists were here to make the next review. Winding around the cubicles as nonchalantly as he could, he did a quick mental roll call. "Evan? Check. Murray? Check. Peg, Keisha, Joanna, Tina, and Charlene? Check. There were a few others, but what Theo considered the "core dream team" were all present and accounted for. He hoped none of them saw the fear in his eyes as he made the quick tour of the floor. When each of them focused on their screens and went to work, Theo made a beeline back to his office to watch from afar. His answer would come soon enough.

Evan went through the established D-MACS scoring sheet to determine the next steps for the COPD'er with sudden onset respiratory failure. He made quick work of the chart and tabbed his calculations based on Jimmy's prior medical history, current presentation, and, to his disdain, his Status Quotient. Jimmy Coltrane's lengthy smoking history combined with his twice divorced, now single status, not to mention being the recipient of unemployment checks for the past three years did not bode well in his favor.

A bead of sweat trickled down Evan's temple as he submitted his scores. He was anxious to see if the changes he had made would work as he hoped. Knowing that prying eyes were most likely closely watching the resulting calculation, he sat and waited for the rest of the panelists to finish their review. He tried to casually lean back so as to see the other panelists but was unable to get a good reading on anyone else. Murray's back was turned to him and all he could hear was his labored breathing, open-mouthed chewing, and lip smacking. None of the other panelists had stood up yet, so he sat and tried to wait patiently. At last, he heard some movement and decided to head to the breakroom to help distract him as he awaited the consolidated feedback response score. A few minutes later, Peg came into the breakroom and grabbed a bottled water.

She whispered over her shoulder to him, "Well, you think it worked?"

Evan ensured no one else was in the room before answering. "I'm not sure yet. I'll check the CFR in a few minutes. Do you think everyone is done? What's taking them so long? This was a slam dunk."

"I know. I know. He would be a sixty-eight using Statis Quotient, don't you think?"

"Definitely. But with the changes I put in, it should have reduced him to a nice thirty-eight or forty-two at worst. I'll know shortly. I'm going to go back to my desk. You wait a couple minutes then go back to your station. I have a contact at dispatch. I'll give him a call after I see the CFR pop up. Let's meet back here in, what, say ten minutes. OK?"

"Got it."

Evan strolled back to his cubicle, whistling this time to add to his nonchalant role-playing.

"Hey Putz, if I wanted to hear some bad whistling, I'd ask for it. Why don't you pipe it down, songbird!"

"Sorry, Murr. You got it."

Evan sat back down, and after another interminable minute or two, the CFR icon was highlighted and ready for review. He clicked on it, double-checking to see if Murray was watching him or not. Murray seemed preoccupied by picking up dropped pretzels off his shirt and popping them back in his mouth.

"Let's see ... let's see. Yes! A sixty-eight!"

"Shut up, will ya?"

"Sorry, Murr. Shutting up now."

As the smacking resumed in Murray's cubical, Evan picked up the phone and called Central Dispatch.

"This is Charles, Central Dispatch."

"Hey Charlie, it's me, Evan. Evan Coleman." He whispered into the receiver hoping to be heard by his old friend but not by anyone else on the floor.

"Evan! My man! How've you been doing? Why are you whispering? Everything OK?"

"Yeah, yeah, just got a slight cold or something. Hey, I was hoping you could do me a quick favor."

"Sure, my brother! What can I do for you?"

"I've been training a bunch of newbies down here at D-MACS and, well, you know how that goes. Good help is hard to find. Anyway, I was hoping to ensure that the case we just sent back to you had the appropriate tablature. Respiratory failure. COPD'er with ..."

"Jimmy. Jimmy Coltrane. Yeah, we got him. Your group gave him a thirty-seven, so we sent him to General Regional. Nothing to it. That sound right to you, Ev?"

"Perfect, Charlie, just perfect. Looks like I trained them right. We got to get together some time again and catch up. Next time, beers are on me!"

"I'm gonna hold you to it! Have a good one, Evan."

Hanging up, Evan smiled to himself. Wasn't it nice when a plan came together?

Theo let out a sigh of relief. He had calculated the patient as well and had come up with a sixty-seven. He was satisfied with the ultimate CFR but pulled up the detail screen to see what the range of scores were on the floor. He was dismayed to see several panelists had given this patient scores in the thirties. Unfortunately, the limitations of the review were blinded and he was unable to see which panelist scored what. This was a D-MACS decision made years ago so as to allow panelists the ability to give honest scores without fear of retaliation. This severely limited Theo's ability to isolate which panelists would have been foolish enough to give such a low score. He decided to go back to the floor to get some feedback from those present to see if he could get anyone to confess. Before he could leave his office, his phone rang.

"This is Theodore Butler. How may I help you?"

"You've got a problem, Theo."

"Um, Samantha! So good to hear from you!" Theo lied in response. "Whatever do you mean?"

"Did you look at the scoring for the patient just now?"

"Yes ma'am, I did. A solid sixty-eight. I reviewed the chart myself and gave a similar score. Everyone seems to be right in line."

"Not everyone. Did you check out the detail screen of the CFR?"

"Well, yeah. I mean, a few scores were low, but they didn't alter the overall aggregate. I'm not sure who did that, but I was just about to go ask around."

"At my level, I can unblind the CFR. Let's see … it's employee number 43776."

Theo instantly recognized Murray's assigned employee number. "Well, um yes, that's one of our long-standing panelists. He's a solid reviewer. A little rough around the edges though dependable on his scoring. Why?"

"He gave the patient a thirteen."

"Thirteen! Well, that must be some mistake. He would never have done such a thing, I can assure you."

"Are you telling me I'm wrong, Theo?"

Theo stammered, "Oh no, no ma'am. I just, well, I mean he's not one to give anyone a break. He's actually been known to be a little *too* harsh on his scoring in the past, if you know what I mean. Not one to low ball anyone."

"Theo. Have a talk with 43776. Or I will."

Click.

Staring at the CFR, Theo hung up the phone. He had no idea that higher-ups could unblind the CFR. As he rose from his desk to go speak with Murray, his phone rang again. Theodore Butler would sometimes go days, no weeks, without any phone calls at all. Now two phone calls back-to-back?

"This is Theodore Butler. How may I help you?"

"Young Theodore! Just the person I wanted to speak with. Let's talk about the latest patient review, shall we?"

Theo sat back down at his desk, confused as to the sudden interest in panelist reviews of late. First Samantha. Now the medical director was calling? It was almost too much for him to handle. As he listened to Dr. Thompkins rattle on, he realized a battle was playing out in the D-MACS world that was over his head and more than his brain could conceptualize. But he knew one thing.

He was going to have to have a little sit down with Murray. Hopefully he would take the critique of his scoring with an open mind and a willingness to improve.

Theo shook his head. After all, this was Murray we are talking about here.

Samantha waited after telling Dotty why she was there. Her nerves were a little frazzled and she hoped she could give Earl the answers to whatever he had summoned her for.

Dotty kept her eyes trained on her as she used the intercom. "Mr. Yarborough, I have a Samantha McAllister here to see you."

The response was quick. "Thanks, Dotty. Yes, please see her in."

Dotty led Samantha to the door and opened it, ushering her through.

"Hello, Mr. Yarborough. You asked to see me?" she asked as Dotty closed the door behind her.

"Oh yes, Samantha. Please, come in and have a seat. I need some information and clarity as to the next steps with this, um, 'beta testing site' you have been overseeing. Where does it stand? Is it ready for prime time? I have several parties interested in knowing the 'ifs' and 'whens' to this." Steepling his fingers on the desk, he leaned forward. "I've been blowing smoke up their ass long enough that it's coming out of their ears. Now they want something tangible. Are we ready to spread this thing to a bigger region? Or, dare I say, nationwide? You've been dragging your feet on this, you know. I need to know where we stand." His expression was a cross between anticipation and frustration. And it was not wasted on Samantha.

She smiled, remembering to crinkle her eyes a little. "I'm so glad you asked, sir. I feel we are closer than ever to get this initiative to go, well, nationwide! It's looking good, really, really good," she lied to the CEO. She hoped the most recent conversation with Theodore Butler would be enough to send this newest change across the goal line. Her most recent meeting with Earl, however, made her decide to be more honest than she would have preferred. "To be totally transparent, however, I think you should know there *has* been a hiccup recently, but I can assure you I have personally addressed it. In fact, I just got off the phone with our beta test site before I came in here, and their latest numbers are in line with my expectations. I have a good feeling about this."

Face now blank, Earl stared at Samantha without saying a word. She knew the game and stared back without breaking the awkward silence.

Finally, Earl caved. "Well, then. That's what I wanted to hear. So, what do you think, say maybe next week we get the team together and develop the strategy for the nationwide launch? I need a timeline, Sam. And it needs to be soon. Next week sound good to you?"

Samantha swallowed hard, hoping to not reveal her uncertainty due to not having all panelists in line. She felt confident she had gotten the medical directors taken care of and, apparently, the shift supervisor as well. However, she had one last hurdle left to ensure complete success.

She couldn't really say anything else, so ... "One more week would be plenty of time, sir. I say go ahead and schedule the meeting, and I'll be ready to present the initiative to the rest of the D-MACS leadership."

Smiling, Earl sat back in his oversized leather desk chair and gave a relieved sigh. His eyes wandered to the side of his desk, and she tracked them to a stack of mail on his desk. An issue of "Yachts and You" lay on the top of his pile. He swung his attention back to her. "That would be terrific, Sam, just terrific. OK then, thanks for seeing me on such short notice."

When Earl was ready to end a meeting, apparently he was ready to end a meeting. He motioned toward the door with a nod of his head.

As Samantha exited, she turned back and asked, "Should I leave your office door open, or closed, sir?"

"Closed, please. Thanks. I have some important work to take care of."

She was quick to notice the yacht catalogue already open on his desk as she tugged on the door handle. As she walked past Dotty's desk, she caught their intercom conversation.

"Yes, Mr. Yarborough."

"Dotty, hold all my calls for now. I need some time to, er, review some reports."

"Yes, Mr. Yarborough."

"Thanks, Dotty."

"Yes, Mr. Yarborough."

Samantha feigned a smile all the way back to her own office. Once there, she closed the door and beelined to her mini wine refrigerator, a scowl replacing the smile. This was a foreign concern for Sam, the possibility of being unsuccessful in any form or fashion. She was determined to not let a few bleeding-heart panelists be a blemish on her track record. She needed a plan that would solidify her hard work.

After pouring herself a healthy amount of a pinot noir, she sat back down at her desk and waited for the resveratrol to get her creative juices flowing. It had never let her down before. Staring at the color and consistency of the burgundy liquid, she thought about the actions she had already taken to shore up potential opposition to her success. Smiling at her reflection in the windowpane, she took another sip of wine and considered her options.

Perhaps her focus was not granular enough, having given all of her attention to leadership. Sip. Maybe it was time to get some direct messaging out to the actual panelists since her efforts thus far had provided inconsistent results. Sip. But how? Who? Sip. Sip. It hit her before she even got to the bottom of her glass. The next step to get the beta test site in line and ready to be transitioned to a nationwide reality should be fun.

"Yeah. That'll do it," Samantha said to her reflection, reapplying her lipstick. She then picked up the phone and made her next crucial call.

TAKING CARE OF BUSINESS

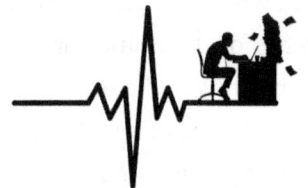

CHAPTER SEVENTEEN

Theodore Butler did not like conflict. As a nonconsequential shift supervisor, he had been moderately successful thus far in his career by just coasting. He liked to think that his panelists respected his "hands off" approach to leadership, never ruffling any feathers or making any waves. While he made an appearance now and then, he preferred to allow the panelists to have the freedom to work at their own style and pace. In fact, Theo had farmed out many of his supervisory tasks to people who were eager to accept more responsibility, freeing up his time to avoid others as much as possible.

Gina, for example, didn't seem to mind reviewing time-cards and submitting payroll variances every other week. Though Theo suspected she was gunning for his job at some point, he could never confirm it. Anyway, she did a much better job at overseeing payroll than Theo ever could. In fact, the complaints from the panelists went from seemingly every paycheck down to zero. All Theo had to do was log in once Gina indicated that all of the pay stubs were correct and ready for processing and click on "Submit." Technically, this was to be done with the scrutiny of the shift supervisor. Since he'd shared his password with Gina years ago, she was able to log on as Theo and get the job done efficiently and accurately.

Same with onboarding and panelist tablature formulas. Having Evan handle the minutiae of these important tasks was another stroke of genius on Theo's part. Evan had an eye for detail and seemed to also relish in the responsibility. Again, technically this was to be done with Theo's oversight. But who had the time, right? He'd given Evan his password years ago, so he was able to take care of any new hire registration in the system as well as any needed changes to formulas running in the background of the panelists' databases.

Theo wasn't even sure if he, himself, could do these tasks anymore as he had never been one hundred percent confident that he ever did them right in the first place. Theo had delegated other responsibilities over the years—so many, in fact, that for the most part he had lost track of which panelist had oversight of what. He was pretty sure Roger ordered office supplies for the floor. And wasn't it Kimberley who arranged all interoffice celebrations (birthdays, work anniversaries, etc.)? And somebody had recently upgraded all the phones in the department. Nice phones. Like, ones with touchscreens and call forwarding and such. Theo made a mental note to try and figure out who had ordered these as they looked expensive and he might get asked about it by someone higher up.

If only Theo could get someone to handle disciplinary action. He had made it through (barely) the crucial conversation with Murray recently about using dating apps while on the job. Now this. And from Samantha, no less.

"Well, no, I haven't had a chance to talk to him yet. After you called, Dr. Thompkins called, basically telling me the same thing. I can assure you, I am going to provide one-on-one education with this panelist about his scoring."

"Training? Are you kidding me? This is bigger than some remediation through extra training. I want you to fire him!"

Theo sat up straight in his chair as the heat of conflict radiated throughout his body. "I can't just fire him, Ms. McAllister," he stammered. "He's got a perfect work performance review for the last, well, since forever." Theo had pulled up Murray's annual evaluations, which were done by Carol. She had given him an "exceptional performance" score (under Theo's login and password, of course). She had even added positive feedback comments as if she were Theo.

"Ahem, I gave him a great review just, well, three months ago." Theo was reading the latest evaluation for the first time. "Some of my comments for him included, 'A real gem of a panelist,' 'Our ace up our sleeve,' and (gulp!) 'Without him, I'm not sure how D-MACS would survive.'" (*Really, Carol?!? I have got to get another panelist to do this for me. Good grief!*).

"I don't care if you said this panelist was the second coming! I'm telling you, Theo, your 'ace up your sleeve' scored the most recent patient a thirteen while most everyone else gave him high sixties as we expected. Fire him!"

"Wait, wait, wait. Please ... give me a chance here. What if I suspend him? How about that? Swift. Bold. Gets your message across loud and clear but gives him room to grow. How about that? Hmmm?" Theo hoped he didn't sound too desperate.

A long pause came across the phone line.

As Theo nervously awaited an answer, he dabbed the sweat off his brow with his shirt sleeve. "Hello? Ms. McAllister? Would, um, would that be acceptable?"

After another long pause, Samantha finally replied. "If suspending him doesn't work, then it will be YOU who will be fired. Do you hear me, Mr. Butler?"

"Yes, ma'am. Loud and clear. This will do the trick, yes ma'am, I just know it will. Thank you, Ms. McAllister. Thank you, thank you, tha—"

Click.

Theo stared at the phone receiver. Apparently, Samantha had nothing else to say, which was just fine by him. He was relieved the conversation had ended, however abruptly. His sense of relief turned to dread as he realized he was going to have to meet with Murray. Again.

"Why haven't I gotten someone else to do this for me yet?" Theo asked as he walked out of his office to retrieve Murray. This was going to be rough and Theo headed towards Murray's station full of dread.

"Why'd it have to be Murray?"

Evan and Peg strolled through the newest surrealism art exhibit at the art museum "for a limited time on loan from the National Archives." Several were from artists they had never heard of, but one name they both recognized and made them stop in their tracks. Salvador Dali. *The Persistence of Memory.*

Evan stood in front of it, mesmerized. A tap on his shoulder startled him from his reverie.

"Evan? Are you OK?"

"This is ... I don't know—this is, like, amazing!"

The two stood for a few silent minutes, staring at the melting watches on the Spanish landscape. Evan had prided himself for never "getting" art. As he had explained to Peg, he came here to think because there was nothing to distract him. This painting, however, made Evan reconsider his unblemished track record of never appreciating any art. Any. The fluidity of the painting and the feeling he got was one he had never experienced before.

"Evan Coleman. Are you becoming an art snob right before my eyes?"

Evan, fixated on the painting, didn't respond.

"Evan? Hello?" Peg waved her hand between Evan's eyes and the painting.

Finally, he turned to Peg, dazed, with a big smile on his face. "I have never felt this way about art. Ever. Wow. That's all I can say. It's like, sometimes I think time has stood still, and this—to me anyway—is what it looks like to me when I get that feeling. Am I making any sense?"

"Perfect."

After a few more minutes, Evan felt he had gotten his fill, and the two of them strolled some more. However, he was still in another world. Not until they got past the Dali exhibit did he feel he'd landed back on planet Earth.

"So. How do you think it went today? As expected? Feeling good?" Peg nudged his arm with her shoulder.

"I think it went about as well as it could go. I mean despite us giving him similar high scores, the patient went directly to the hospital, even though Status Quotient would have normally kicked him to the curb." He furrowed his brow. Something felt off.

"What's wrong?" said Peg. "That's good, right? Exactly what we're trying to do?"

"Well, yes. Only—while I can't see the direct scores by panelists, I did see some pretty low ones. Like, really low. It might be a problem. When I get back, I need to elevate the coefficient on their tablature a smidge so as to not set off any alarms. Other than that, I think it went like clockwork."

Peg smiled and leaned into Evan with her arm intertwined in his. "I knew you could do it! And it feels like we are doing the right thing, doesn't it? At least from my perspective it does. I just hope no one on our floor gets in trouble for it. You don't think anyone is going to get in trouble, do you?"

She let go of Evan's arm and stared at a painting of a leg on fire. Or a tree limb in the sunlight. Evan couldn't tell.

"No one is going to get in trouble, Peg. Trust me on this. I don't think anyone can see which panelists scored what, so it is blinded in our favor. To be extra cautious though, when we get back, I think I should reset the input tabulation formula, to ensure no one's scores will get them in any sort of trouble. Also, I'll check in with Dr. Thompkins to see if there is anything on his end that I need to address. We're heading in a good direction. And, yes. We *are* doing the right thing. I can feel it. Just one more thing before we head back, though." Evan looked at Peg with what he hoped were pleading doe eyes.

Peg stopped walking. "What is it? Are you feeling okay? You look queasy all of a sudden."

"What? No! Can we go back and look at the melting clocks one more time?"

Theo was not good with confrontations. Nor was he that stellar with providing coaching. But he truly reached new levels of incompetence with issuing discipline. He had the terrible idea of quietly telling Murray he was being suspended at his cubicle. He realized his mistake the moment Murray raised his voice, wishing he had the good sense to have done this in the safe confines of his office.

"Suspended? For what, Theo? I haven't done anything wrong! I swear! This is the Murr-man, you're talking to, you know? I demand to know what I have done. Tell me!"

Several of Murray's co-workers raised their heads over their cubicle dividers to see what the commotion was all about. "Let's talk about it in my office, Murray," Theo said in a loud whisper, hoping to de-escalate the rapidly increasing volume of defiance. It didn't work.

Standing up, Murray proceeded to knock some papers and pens onto the floor. Following Theo towards his office, he continued his defense. "Tell me, Theo! This makes no sense!"

Ignoring Murray, Theo kept walking toward his office. Once Murray came in, he closed the door, the entire floor of panelists still craning their necks in their direction.

"Please. Have a seat."

"I'll stand. I have not been on any more dating websites. I have not approached any of my female co-workers. I've done every damn thing you've asked, Theo. What is this about?"

Heat rose up Theo's shirt collar, perspiration prickling

on his upper lips and under each arm. "Yes, yes, I have noticed and I truly appreciate that, Murray. You have done great on that front. Thank you."

"Well, if it isn't that, what is it?"

Theo decided to add some context so as to take the direction of anger off of him and more towards upper management. "As you know, we've been under a lot of scrutiny of late regarding our scoring of patients utilizing Status Quotient. As the beta testing site, all eyes are on us to see how well it works in, um, improving the numbers, so to speak, of our chart reviews."

"Yeah? And?"

New beads of sweat broke out on Theo's forehead and the back of his neck. The circle of moisture under each arm expanded exponentially in diameter.

"The, um, most recent patient review submission? Well, um, you seemed to score him lower than anyone else. Like, a lot lower. And, um, that sorta caught the eye of some of those in, um, in upper management and they— honestly, this isn't coming from me, you gotta believe me—it's upper admin. They, well, they said I needed to suspend you for it."

Murray sat down as several wet locations on Theo's shirt bloomed. He shook his head. "Not your, decision, huh? Came straight from upper administration? That's it then. How long am I suspended?"

Theodore Butler had never issued a suspension before and hadn't bothered to review the policy of D-MACS for this level of punishment. Rather than appear unprepared, he just guessed. "The rest of the week. With pay. Then, when you come back on Monday, we will go over a chart or two together to ensure we are on the same page. Sound good?"

As today was Thursday, Murray felt a three-day weekend actually sounded pretty good to him. He knew the policy for D-MACS stipulated a five-day suspension without pay, but he didn't bother to correct Theo. Murray got up, knowing that Theo was being strong armed by someone higher than him. And he had a sneaky suspicion that Evan Coleman had something to do with it. Theo was just a pawn and, for some unknown reason, Murray was the patsy. "I understand, Theo. We'll talk Monday. Thanks for letting me know, and I look forward to working with you next week on this."

Theo opened and closed his mouth a few times, his expression showing clear surprise. Murray guessed he'd expected a fight. No sense in that with a mini vacation on the horizon. He left Theo, who'd collapsed in his chair with a relieved sigh, and didn't look back.

Murray went to his cubicle and shut down his computer and grabbed his keys and jacket. He could feel Evan staring at him and spun to address him. "What are you looking at, Putz? I'm leaving for the day. You got a problem with that?"

Evan, like the rest of the panelists, would have heard Murray yelling at Theo as they walked to Theo's office. Specifically, he would have heard the word "suspension." Murray had expected Evan's dumb face to be full of gloating. Instead, his forehead was puckered and he was gnawing on his lip. Was he worried?

"No, Murr. Hey, everything, um, OK? You all good?"

Suspecting Evan had something to do with all this, Murray leaned in, narrowing his eyes. "You tell me, Putz. You've been all chummy with Peg and several others—you got something to tell me?" Murray hoped Evan would give some context as to what was going on and, perhaps, show his hand in the suspension.

"Oh, nothing going on around here, Murr, you know that. Another day in dullsville, right?"

Evan's quick denial was confirmation that he was up to something. Murray just couldn't figure out what, and Evan didn't seem like he would give an inch.

"Well, then ..." Evan drew out the word. "When will you be back?"

"Monday, not that it's any of your business."

"Oh, OK. Well, enjoy your long weekend, Murr."

Just then, Theo rounded on the floor, making small talk with various panelists. He was not very conspicuous to his real intent, as Murray assumed he was there to ensure that he would leave the floor.

Murray growled at Evan and made a beeline to the elevator. Avoiding the other panelists' stares, he left the floor without any further conversation. He was determined to find out what was going on with Evan and the others and how he got pinned as the scapegoat for their suspicious activity. As the elevator doors closed, he noticed Evan and Peg eyeing each other with concerned expressions. This was further confirmation for Murray that these two were up to something—and he was going to get to the bottom of it.

After all, this was the Murr-man they were dealing with.

Making his way around with his white hand towel, Harry wiped the wood to a bright glisten under the bar lights. He used this time to check in with each customer as well, offering up a refill or a sympathetic ear. His instincts were well-honed over the years, and he was able to discern the needs of each patron, many times before they even uttered their first syllable. Harry felt that, in a small way, he had the opportunity to be an important part of someone's life during their lowest moments. He was careful not to offer up too much in the way of solutions, instead, allowing the loquacious lamenters ample opportunity to figure out their next steps on their own. Harry joked that his happy hour pricing was far less expensive than some uptown therapist's upcharges.

"He's scum. That's all there is to it. Scum of the earth, I tell ya."

"Sounds like it. Pure scum."

"But he's not scum! How could you say that? He's the salt of the earth, and I'm the fool. It's me, don't you see? It's my fault. I pushed him too hard!"

"I wonder what you could do to get him back?" Harry offered up, suppressing a yawn.

"I tell ya. (Hiccup). I'm gonna go back to him and make this right. He's probably sitting there, right now, wondering where I am. (Crying starts). I'm going to fix him his favorite dinner and tell him how sorry I am. That's what I'll do. I mean, how could I not see it? Scum? Harrumph. You don't know him like I know him, Harry. I'm gonna make this right. You'll see."

Harry knew she wasn't going to make this right.

He had never kidded himself in his success rate. A good listener knew when the time was right to set someone on a new course and when to let someone learn from their mistakes. No matter how many times they made the same blunders in their relationships.

"See you next week, Harry."

"See you, Doreen."

After all, some people seemed to never learn.

Moving on around the bar, Harry stopped his polishing in front of a new face. He had ordered a gin and tonic about twenty minutes prior but hadn't even had a sip yet. Honestly, the poor guy looked a little unhinged and unpredictable, and, well, smelled a little unbathed.

"Why the long face, mister? Can't be that bad, can it?"

Harry had a sixth sense of how to open up closed off faces.

"I'd rather not talk about it. Can't I just sit here in peace? Jeez. It's still America last time I checked."

Shrugging, Harry made the rounds again. After about fifteen minutes, he found himself cleaning the same spot in front of long-faced Gin-and-Tonic. Which was still untouched.

Humming offkey, Harry slowly wiped the bar with his towel. Most times, just being in the proximity of someone can get them to open up. Although it happened quite rarely, Harry's been known to be wrong before.

"Is this the treatment you give all your customers who want to sit quietly with their own thoughts?"

"Lady trouble? Been there, done that, buddy. I mean, don't get me started."

Gin-and-Tonic returned Harry's inquiry with a scowl and a low growl.

"No? Gotta be money woes. Let me tell you, that's my middle name. I know it's a funny middle name, but, hey, I wasn't able to cast a vote when my mom and dad named me, you know? Harry 'Money Woes' Coleman. You know what I mean?"

This time, the scowl and growl were accompanied by an eye roll.

"It's something at work. I tell you, I knew it when you walked in here and ordered the gin and tonic. I was just joshin' about the lady troubles and money woes. Of course it's trouble at the ol' salt mine. Could have seen it for miles."

Harry's persistence paid off. The slight rise in the eyebrows, while subtle, was just enough for an expert like Harry to perceive. Of course, ninety-nine percent of the time, it was going to be trouble with a spouse, trouble with money, or trouble with work. That was just the law of averages for ya.

"I'd rather not talk about it."

Taking a gamble, Harry made a safe bet that this one was going to be complaining about being unfairly singled out on the job. He decided to bait the hook. "Oh sure, sure, I understand. Wouldn't blame you if I were in your shoes. I tell you though, if it were me being blamed for something I didn't do, I'd be pretty down in the dumps about it as well. But, hey. That's just me."

Harry polished the bar slightly away from Gin-and-Tonic. He worked the towel while humming to himself even more offkey, this time a bit more quietly, as if to himself.

Harry then returned, as if he had missed a spot, sensing Gin-and-Tonic might open up.

"I mean, I do my job better than any of the half-wits they got working there, and *I'm* the one who gets in trouble?"

Not wanting to press for details, he decided to let him open up on his own terms. "Let me get you a fresh drink. The one in front of you is just about all melted ice."

He quickly prepared another gin and tonic and placed it in front of the forlorn, dejected employee.

"Thanks."

"Where was it you said you work?" He hadn't said, but Harry thought it would pry him open a bit more.

"Government job. I work for D-MACS."

"D-MACS, huh? My nephew works down there as well. He does something with computers, but I'm not exactly sure what."

As if on cue, Evan entered the Hideaway, stopping about halfway to the bar when his eyes landed on Gin-and-Tonic.

Seriously? Here? Evan gave an internal groan.

Why'd it have to be Murray?

"Well, lookie, lookie, if it isn't ol' jerkface." Murray could always be counted on to not hide his feelings.

"Oh, um, hey Murray. Haven't seen you here before." Evan slowly made his way to the bar, sitting a couple of barstools away from him.

"Houlihan's Hideaway—where friends go to let it all unwind!" Harry, always the diplomat, dipped his head and strolled away, giving Evan and Murray space. Evan noted, however, that he remained in the vicinity. Just in case. In the background, Harry hummed.

Murray glared at Evan then turned back to his drink, sulking.

"Listen, Murray. I feel like I need to explain some things. I think there's an off chance that I, um, got you ... suspended. And I feel terrible about it."

Murray slowly turned toward Evan. "I *knew* it! I knew you and your precious little Peg had something to do with it!"

"Now, Murray, let's leave Peg out of it. She had absolutely nothing to do with it. But, please, let me explain. Will ya?"

Murray continued to glare at Evan.

"You gotta believe me, Murr. I didn't realize anyone would get hurt by my experiment. I've already changed it back. But can I buy you a drink and try to explain?"

Murray pointed to his full gin and tonic and pantomimed the word, "Duh!"

"OK, well then, um, how about we just go sit over there at one of the booths, and I'll go over everything with you. I think if you'll hear me out, you'll not only understand but also be motivated to make some changes like me."

"Listen, Putz. There isn't really anything you could say to change my mood. I come in to work, I do my job, I enter a few scores on a few patients, then I clock out. Except, noooooooo, not today. Today I got weed wacked for just keeping my head down and doing the right thing. So, thanks, but no thanks."

"Murr. I understand you are ticked off, and rightly so. I mean, I would be if I were in your shoes. If you'll let me, though, I can fill you in on what exactly's happening around here. And it isn't pretty."

Murray got up from his barstool and grabbed his drink.

"I'll give you five minutes. That's it, Putz."

"That's all I'll need. Thanks, Murray. Come on."

The two of them walked over to one of the empty booths lining each side of the bar. Evan caught Harry's eye as they sat down, giving a nod to indicate things were heading in the right direction. In return, Harry winked and tapped near the outside corner of his open eye, indicating he would keep watch from the bar.

Evan started to explain, but Murray interrupted.

"Listen here. I don't really care what you have to say. I don't like you. You don't like me. Fine. You've always been jealous of me, which is understandable. But from now on, you and little Peg need to keep me and my work out of your pet projects. I do my job, and I do it damn well. Whatever hair-brained scheme you're up to, that ain't my business. Just make sure you stay away from me and let me be Murray. You understand?" Murray looked at the door and checked his watch.

"Murr. C'mon, man. Please let me explain. This was all unintentional. I had no idea anyone higher up would be watching over our shoulders. I seriously—"

"I don't care, Evan. Nothing you can say would make me see your side. Just keep me out of it from now on. I will tell you this though—if you cross me again, I'll report you so fast your head will spin. I bet ol' Theo would just looooove to know what you and your group of losers have been up to." Murray continued to divide his attention between Evan and the front entrance to the bar.

"But Murray—"

"I'm done." Murray sat up straight and slid from the booth. "Besides, my date just walked in. I have bigger fish to fry, Evan. So stay out of my way, got it?"

Murray walked toward the door. Straining to see who his date was, Evan had to lean out of his side of the booth. She looked familiar, but he couldn't place her.

"Well, that could have gone better. What was I thinking? You can't reason with Murray."

Just then Harry came over. "You two resolve your differences?"

"He's crazy, Harry. I mean, while I didn't have huge expectations of getting him to understand things, I did hope he would at least have the decency to listen to me. Oh well, he is who he is."

"Hey, the lady who just came in and is now sitting with your work friend. Isn't she the same lady who you and I spoke to not too long ago? Back when you were all fretful about your job and what you were being asked to do?"

Evan froze. He knew exactly who Murray's blind date was. "Harry. I need you to get me out of here, out the back entrance. Can you distract them? I'll explain later."

"I'm on it."

As Harry burst into the first verse of "Hello, Young Lovers," he wandered over to Murray and his date. Evan eased out past the bar and into the back area of Houlihan's, unseen. He paused and turned back to Murray. He could see that his date, Samantha McAllister, was already studying the bar and eyeing the front door as Harry started with the chorus.

Good ol' Harry. Evan left the bar through the back entrance, eager to call Peg to tell her of Murray and his latest escapades. Good ol' Harry and good ol' Murray. Well, Samantha was getting what she deserved.

AS IT IS WRITTEN, SO IT SHALL BE DONE

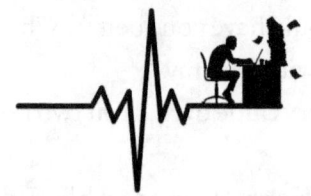

CHAPTER EIGHTEEN

Evan dialed Peg as soon as he got outside. He still couldn't believe what he'd just seen, and knew she'd be gob-smacked as well. He was not mistaken.

"Wait, what? Murray and Samantha?"

"I know! Can you believe it? Surely she had no idea who he was. I'm telling you, Peg. Those dating sites are just terrible. I wish I were a fly on the wall. Don't you?"

"Well ... why can't we be? I'm not too far away from Houlihan's right now. Wanna go spy?"

"Peg! That's ... well ... that's a great idea! Listen, meet me on the corner before you get to Harry's place, and we can go in through the back entrance. This is gonna be good."

Hanging up, Evan smiled. Peg was more adventurous than he gave her credit for, and she pushed him beyond his normal self-imposed limits. She was the constant in all of this, the one who gave him the confidence he oftentimes lacked. He was glad he was going to get to see her again. Evan made his way to the corner of 17th and Maple and waited for Peg to arrive. After a few minutes, he saw Peg hurrying toward him, a mischievous smile on her face.

He returned her smile with an even bigger grin. Evan greeted her. "Hey, 007. Are you ready to spy on the most disastrous pairing ever dreamed up?"

"It's Bond. James Bond, if you please." Giggling, Peg grabbed Evan's hand. "Where is this back entrance?"

"C'mon." He took her hand, tugged her around the corner, and led the way up the back alley toward the rear entrance to Houlihan's Hideaway. Once inside, they wound their way through stacks of boxes. He almost knocked over Harry as they turned the corner of the supply room.

Grabbing his chest, Harry laughed. "You two scared the dickens out of me! You gotta let a guy know when you are going to break into his establishment and give him a heart attack! What are you two sneaks up to?"

They both placed their index fingers to their lips at the same time.

"Shhh, Harry," said Evan. "We came back to see that guy I work with and his date. How is it going?"

Harry laughed again, immediately covering his mouth, thus containing the volume.

"Not good. Not good at all. Apparently, he met her on some dating app. She yelled it a couple times. What was it? Oh, shoot. It was … no, it was"—Harry snapped his fingers— "Oh yeah! 'Millionaire Mingle'. She kept yelling at him that he obviously lied about his profile and she should have had better sense when he had asked to meet her at this dump. Can you believe it? Houlihan's? A dump? I mean, the nerve of her!"

Craning his head, Evan asked, "Are they still here? We gotta see this!"

Harry took a few steps toward the bar and peered around the corner. "Yep. But you two better hurry. She's got her purse and coat in her hands. Here, let me help you two sleuths." Harry slid a few boxes around and pulled the curtain separating the front of the bar from the back storage area. "There. I better make my rounds."

As Harry returned to work, Evan and Peg positioned themselves to watch the drama. Based on Evan's observations, a second date would not be forthcoming.

"I can't believe it." Samantha didn't even bother to keep her voice down. "I'm putting in a complaint with Millionaire Mingle. They have gotta vet the bank accounts of the guys out there. I can't believe I wasted my evening on the likes of you!"

"Say, listen here, lady. You aren't exactly my type either, you know what I mean? I mean, the face, it's OK. You could stand to use a little less eye shadow, but by and large, you aren't *that* bad looking, you know what I'm saying? Not the best, not the worst. Why, when you came in, I thought you were pretty enough, enough to make up for the lack of curves in the ol' booty department. But, hey, that's just me. I'm a generous guy."

She set down her coat and purse, grabbed a mostly empty glass of wine, drained it, and grabbed her belongings again. Evan was fascinated.

"You are absolutely the crudest pig I've ever met." Her words slurred a little.

Focused on her empty wine glass, Murray landed one more parting shot. "Oh, hey, a little advice. On the first date, maybe ease up on the wine swigging. What, you had three glasses in all of fifteen minutes? Seems a little desperate."

"ARRGH! GOODBYE!"

Samantha turned heels and stumbled up the few stairs to the door. As the door closed, Harry made his way to the booth.

"Well, I guess that's it, huh, mister?"

Looking up at Harry, Murray shrugged. "It's hard to find a good woman out here, you know? Good grief! I'd say I dodged the ol' bullet with that piece of work. Anyways, I'll take the check."

"You still didn't touch your gin and tonic. And she had three glasses of wine? How about this? Twenty bucks and let's call it even. No need to go into debt over a bad romance."

Murray pulled a twenty dollar bill out of his pocket and found two quarters as well for a tip. "Here you go. Thanks."

Harry stared at the two quarters in his hands as Murray left the bar, whistling "Bad Romance" by Lady Gaga. Once he was safely out, Evan and Peg made their way over to where Harry stood.

"Fifty cents. Big tipper, that friend of yours."

"Oh, he isn't our friend, Harry. Not even close. Thanks for letting us watch the fireworks, though. Hey, since the booth is open, how about a couple of drinks for me and Peg? And this time, I'm paying, you hear me?"

As Evan and Peg settled into the booth, Harry walked back to the bar, singing off key as always.

Good ol' Harry.

Watching the smoke rings as they burst apart on the ceiling, Dr. Thompkins thought about his next move. His watch showed him it was now past nine in the morning, and the day shift panelists should be making their way onto the floor. He decided to take a chance and dialed the number.

"D-MACS, this is Evan. How may I direct your call?"

"Evan! Just the panelist I was hoping to talk to. How are you, young man?"

Evan spoke in a hushed tone. "Um, good, good, Dr. Thompkins. How can I help you?"

"Well, I was just sitting here thinking about our last conversation at your uncle's fine establishment and wanted to see how things are progressing. Any news?"

Evan's voice grew distant, and a chair or something squeaked in the background before he returned to the phone. "Sorry, had to make sure no one can hear me. So, yeah, though. A lot has gone on. Yesterday was crazy, absolutely crazy. We made the changes to the"—he whispered even lower—"input tabulation and before you know it, one of my coworkers got suspended. All because of the change I had put in. I mean, I don't want anyone to get hurt around here, Dr. Thompkins. So I changed the formula back. I can't lose my job, you hear me?"

Taking a slow drag on the pipe, Dr. Thompkins considered this. "Well, if the formula is changed back, won't it just go back to how Samantha and the rest want the scores to be? This isn't good."

"Agreed, but I don't know what to do at this point. I say we wait until some of the smoke clears, don't you think?"

"I'm afraid time isn't our friend here, young man. Earl Yarborough wants this to go nationwide as soon as next week! He seems to believe that the kinks have been worked out and wants to spread it across the nation. We have got to make a drastic change and make it now, Evan. We have no time to waste."

Evan let out a groan. "And here I was feeling bad because of Murray. This is even worse. What should I do, Dr. Thompkins? I can't risk changing the scores now. Not knowing that the higher ups can see the numbers."

"OK. Listen to me. I am one of the so-called 'higher ups' as you describe it, you know. I saw the scoring that caused your co-worker to get suspended. And so did Samantha, I suspect. But we can only see your employee numbers, not names. Go ahead and get your group to score without Status Quotient for now, and let me run interference with her, okay? Since young Theo doesn't have the same detailed access Samantha and I have, we are the only ones who can really see the scoring details. I'll distract Samantha until Monday. But then, we are going to need to get drastic."

"Sounds good. You sure you can keep Samantha from looking at the details? I mean, if I get canned, I'll be mad— but not as upset as if some of the others get fired over it. Especially Peg, you know?"

As the smoke plume rose above his head, Dr. Thompkins reassured Evan. "Trust me, young man. This isn't my first rodeo, believe it or not. My distraction should hold her for a few days. That will give me time over the weekend to come up with the coup de grâce that is needed to end this once and for all. This has gone too far. And I for one am not going to let some bureaucrat dictate how I deliver health care. I tell you, Evan, this ends on Monday. Good day!"

After hanging up the phone, Dr. Thompkins got up from his desk and paced back and forth. He hoped he had convinced Evan that he could find a solution. Running his hand through the remaining hairs on his head, he worried if the answer would actually come to him. First step, however, was to stall Samantha. Rummaging through the papers on his desk, he found the memo that he hoped would assist in his efforts to divert her attention, albeit briefly. He jotted down a few notes then picked up the phone. As he gazed up at the ceiling, he was reminded of his younger Catholic upbringing and said a quick prayer to Saint Jude Thaddeus, the patron saint of desperate situations. He was going to need all the help he could get.

Samantha's phone rang. Instead of chucking it across the room like she wanted, she answered through gritted teeth. "Yes? This had better be good."

"Ms. McAllister! Dr. Thompkins here. I'm so glad I caught you. How are you on this beautiful morning?"

Samantha was still steaming from her disastrous date with Murray the night before and had yet to recover. What a jerk he was!

"Fine. What do you want?" Samantha never liked small talk. This didn't improve when in a foul mood.

"Well, I am so delighted you asked. I'm afraid I have some disconcerting news to review with you if I could spare a few minutes out of your schedule. It's about the roll-out you are proposing for end of next week." Dr. Thompkins's voice was annoyingly chipper for something that sounded like potential bad news.

"What about it? We are rolling out nation-wide next week. Period. I already have the schedule in place, and you, Dr. Thompkins, are slated to lead the mandatory education via video conference. This has been sent out already. What 'disconcerting news' are you referring to?"

"I'm terribly sorry to have to be the one to be the bearer of bad news. I truly am."

"WHAT IS IT, HAROLD?" Samantha shouted into the phone.

"It appears there is a scheduled software update that IT has already on the books, which is going to necessitate a small delay. You know how difficult it is to get them to move these things around. It must have been an oversight. I'm sure if you make a few calls, on the behalf of Earl, you might have better luck. But with this unavoidable update looming, I fear we will not be able to get the Status Quotient algorithm installed on all D-MACS panelists' computers."

"NO ONE TOLD ME ABOUT THIS!" Samantha roared into the phone.

"I'm holding a copy of the memo in my hand right now. It was sent out by IT last month. It probably would have been a benefit had they sent a reminder or something, don't you think? But I bet if you made a few phone calls you could move mountains, Ms. McAllister." Dr. Thompkins coughed in the background. "Terribly sorry about that. Had a tickle in my throat."

"I will NOT delay this roll out. Not a chance. I am calling IT now. There will be NO delay, you hear me? Be prepared for the education as scheduled, do you understand me, Harold?"

"But of course, I plan on reviewing my presentation today and, as you know, am excited to spread this out to the masses, as it were. Please let me know if there is anything I can do to assist you in your crusade!" (Cough, cough).

She made a face. He'd better get that cough under control. No time to get sick now. "I'm perfectly capable of handling a bunch of computer nerds. I mean, how difficult can it be?"

Click. She hung up on him.

Dr. Thompkins burst out laughing—he'd barely been able to stifle it with his fabricated coughing. Samantha was about to encounter the worst headache of her day. It was painfully obvious that she had never dealt with the unmovable, deeply entrenched force of those working in Information Technology at D-MACS. For one, they required every request or change to be done via work order. And secondly, the work orders were all done on paper. And to make it worse, it had to be done in triplicate. The scheduled downtime on Monday could not be altered at this late of a date. Dr. Thompkins thanked the saints for the reprieve. His dwindling faith in Catholicism was, for the moment, restored due to this mini-miracle. What perfect timing! This would only give him a day or two delay, but he was hopeful that he would be able to generate a way to permanently disable the nationwide rollout between now and then.

Come on, Saint Jude. Don't fail me now!

The soul stylings of the saxophonist putting his all into the bluesy rendition of "What a Wonderful World" did little to improve Samantha's mood while on hold. After the fifth cycle of the song, interrupted periodically with a recorded message stating her call was "very important to us, please remain on the line" only made her angrier. Slamming down the phone, she proceeded to spend the rest of the day making multiple phone calls to whomever she thought could help, composing highly inflammatory emails, setting up a task force that would meet to revise the current approval process for computer shutdown scheduling, and finally, in complete and total surrender, filling out a work order. On paper. In triplicate. Once completed and placed in interoffice mail, she decided to break the news to Earl Yarborough that, due to unforeseen circumstances beyond her control, the nationwide roll out of Status Quotient would have to have a slight delay.

As she made her way to the CEO's office, she managed to catch him as he was leaving for the day.

"Earl! Sir! Could I have a quick minute? I know it's late."

Looking at his watch, Earl responded. "Can't this wait, Sam? I have a dinner date I'm going to be late for. It's already after six o'clock."

"I'll walk with you, sir."

As they headed toward the elevators, Samantha proceeded to explain to Earl how his directive to get the beta test site spread to all D-MACS panelists across the country would have to be delayed due to the software update with computer shut down. She braced for impact, expecting to be lambasted with a verbal storm of expletives and imprecations to make her wish to be anywhere but here. To her shock and surprise, however, she was met with a slow laugh that rose to a full chuckle.

"Sam, you really should read your memos closer," Earl said, stepping into the elevator. As the doors began to close, he added, "That software update was last week!"

She could hear him continue to laugh, even after the elevator doors closed.

"ARRRGH!" Samantha shouted. "That son of a bitch!"

Samantha stormed back to her office, furious to have wasted her entire day. She slammed her office door, grabbed a bottle of wine and a glass, and filled it to the rim. There would be no softening the tannins through aeration on this bottle of Petit Verdot. This bottle was for rapid consumption. She gulped the contents without noticing the complex flavors and aromas of plums, dark cherry, and blackberries that had been carefully crafted for the most finicky of wine enthusiasts. She stewed in her fury toward being duped by Dr. Thompkins. NO WAY this was done by accident. He was trying to play her at her own game. How dare this curmudgeon think he could challenge her? As she refilled her glass, her anger intensified. Staring out of her window, she guzzled the contents of the second pouring, ruminating about the turn of events.

"You may have won this battle, doc. But Samantha McAllister ALWAYS wins the war!"

As she poured the remaining contents into her glass, she stared at the dark red liquid and finally gave a faint hint of a smile. When the next steps formulated in her head, she slowed her breathing and regained some level of calm.

"Samantha McAllister always wins her wars."

Gulp.

WHEN PUSH COMES TO SHOVE

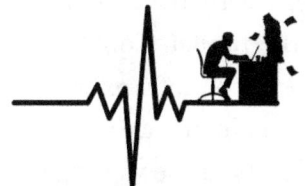

CHAPTER NINETEEN

Bill Wilson rarely saw the inside of Regional General on weekends. As lead evaluator, he stuck to the normal business hours of a Monday-through-Friday work week. Oh, he occasionally received emails and various calls or texts on his off hours, but he had a relatively consistent level of disconnect from the hospital on his off time. This weekend, however, seemed destined to make up for all the years of uninterrupted peace all at once. As soon as he handled one crisis, another call came in. Apparently, no end was in sight to the onslaught of patients arriving at the hospital. Finally, on Sunday afternoon, he felt he needed to see the chaos for himself.

Arriving at the emergency department entrance, he was shocked at the scene before him. Several ambulances were lined up, waiting to deliver more patients. Walking into the hospital, he heard shouts of frustration and helplessness from the doctors and nurses running here and there, at times colliding with each other as if in a Three Stooges short. It would have been comical if it weren't so stressful. Bill found the head emergency physician and was able to stop him to get a real time assessment of the current situation.

"Well, Bill, apparently the dam has broken and we are the short end of the funnel. Look! I have them lined up along the walls, we are out of stretchers, and we had to get some cots from the maintenance guys to create a makeshift M.A.S.H. unit of sorts in the waiting room. Don't get me wrong, I like crazy. That's why I work in the ER. But this is like nothing I've seen before. I hope you got some calvary on speed dial because we need them, like, yesterday." He ran off, barking orders to no one, walking as fast as he could, and doing his best to make a path among the patients who were all around, their hands outstretched as if he were Jesus among the lepers.

Bill stood paralyzed, not knowing what to do. Finally, with no other options, he made the call he really didn't want to make.

"It's terrible, Ms. McAllister, just terrible. No, I'm here in the lobby and I have no idea where all of these patients have come from. Did something change recently that I wasn't made aware of? This can't continue! I'm going to do my best to help out and triage a few of these patients, but I'm not sure how they are going to make it through the night at this rate."

Bill got some much-needed reassurance from Samantha that she was going to "take care of things once and for all." He rolled up his sleeves and joined the weekend evaluator in attempting to screen and triage the various patients who kept rolling in. He was surprised to see the type of patients that were occupying every nook and cranny of the emergency department, many of which he had not seen in a long time. Most of these patients would have never arrived at Regional General in the past. He shook his head, feeling that D-MACS was unraveling before his eyes. As he went from physician to physician to reassure them that administration had been contacted and was taking steps to curtail the onslaught, he realized he was the one who needed the most reassurance. He decided to call Carl to get some night shift assistance.

"Yes sir! I'll be right in. Oh, boy!"

Bill knew that Carl was eager to please and would relish in being needed in this moment of crisis. Once he arrived, the two of them made quick work of screening the patients who had not been vetted. After a few hours, all of the patients had their paperwork taken care of and a glimmer of respite seemed to be in sight.

"I'm heading home for a few hours of sleep. Will you be OK helping out for a little bit tonight?"

Mimicking a soldier's salute, Carl stood at attention. "Sir! Yes, sir!"

Though Bill rolled his eyes, he was glad to have Carl's unabashed dedication to the company. As he left the hospital, Bill noticed no more ambulances were lined up at the moment and felt safe to leave. Getting in his car, he sent up a silent prayer that Samantha was going to work her magic to get things back to normal.

Before arriving at the office Monday morning, Evan stopped at a bakery and purchased two dozen donuts and one bear claw, knowing it was Murray's favorite. He was not ashamed to try and appeal to Murray's sweet tooth, hope-fully to reconcile things with him. As much as he disliked Murray, he knew that he was responsible for his suspension and had an insatiable level of guilt. He hoped today would not be too hectic. He arrived early, when only a few other panelists had gotten there. He placed the boxes of donuts in the breakroom and proceeded to make himself a cup of cof-fee. As he was stirring in the sugar and creamer, he heard a voice from the doorway.

"Well, you'll be glad to know my date was a whack job, Putz. I bet that will put a smile on your stupid face."

Evan, relieved Murray was talking to him, said, "I'm sorry to hear that, Murr. What happened?"

Murray poured a cup of coffee into his "You Don't Have to Be Crazy to Work Here, but It Helps!" coffee mug, com-plete with a picture of a crossed-eyed clown. Murray hadn't rinsed out the cup from last week and was pouring fresh cof-fee into the dirty cup with old, curdled liquid at the bottom. Evan shuddered at Murray's lack of hygiene but did his best to overlook it.

"She was cray-cray, that's what! She made some big deal about saying I hadn't been 'honest'—Murray used air quotes—on my profile on the dating app. I mean, everyone lies on those things, am I right?"

Evan had never used a dating app but felt that going along with him at this point in time was the best tactic to patch things up and seemingly be in alignment.

"Of course! I think mine says I'm six foot three, and my profile picture is Brad Pitt." Evan wasn't sure if dating apps included height and photos but took a gamble.

"See! You get it! Good grief, women out there are just impossible to please, you know what I mean?"

"Definitely, Murr. Women! I mean, you can't live with them and you can't shoot 'em either!" Evan wasn't exactly sure what the phrase meant but had heard it in a movie once and took another chance that Murray would agree with the sentiment.

"So, I did some reflecting this weekend, and I accept your apology. You're a putz and obviously had no idea that whatever hairbrained scheme you were up to would send ol' Murr to the sidelines. Just don't let it happen again, got it?" Murray proceeded to punch Evan in the arm to emphasize his point.

Rubbing his arm, Evan exhaled in relief.

"Of course, of course. And, hey, I just feel terrible. Here. You like bear claws, right?"

Grabbing the pastry, Murray accepted the peace offering.

"Hell yeah, they are the best. Is this from Adleman's?"

"You know it!"

Murray sipped his coffee and then proceeded to do his best to attempt to devour the baked delicacy in one bite.

Chewing open mouthed, Murray said, "Thanks, Putz."

Evan tried not to look as flaky bits flew in a frenzy from Murray's mouth.

"It's gonna be a good day, Murray. Let's do this."

They left the breakroom and headed to their cubicles. Evan turned on his computer, he settled into his office chair and got situated, ready to start the day. As the D-MACS logo slowly came to view on the computer monitor, Evan's phone rang.

"D-MACS, this is Evan. How may I direct your call?"

"Good morning, Evan. I need to fill you in on the weekend and what I am going to need you to do today."

Evan listened to Dr. Thompkins recount the way he had run interference with Samantha McAllister on Friday with the mandatory software upgrade announcement.

"But the upgrade was last week, sir."

"I knew that and you knew that. But *she* didn't!" Dr. Thompkins' laughter on the phone made Evan laugh as well, causing Murray to lean back and tell Evan to "shut the hell up."

"Sorry, Murr, sorry." Evan lowered his voice as he continued his conversation with Dr. Thompkins.

"So … what do we need to do today? Surely she's realized you stalled her by now."

"Oh, and then some. She is royally pissed and, well, I don't know exactly what she has planned, but it isn't going to be good, that's for sure. So I need you to get word out to your fellow panelists to stick to the script today. Use Status Quotient today like your life depends on it. I have a feeling our Ms. McAllister is going to be looking closely over each of your shoulders today to see if things are still awry. You can count on that. Meanwhile, I am going to be pretending like I am going along with the big nationwide rollout this week."

"But sir! That can't happen!"

"I said shut up, Putz! Some of us are trying to work here!"

Having Murray back was, Evan realized, a mixed blessing.

Evan whispered to Dr. Thompkins, "It's a disaster, sir."

"I know, I know, and I have been working with Simon

all weekend to develop a final death blow to this. But you must trust me on this. Fly straight and narrow today. More to come. I'm counting on you, son."

"Yes, sir. I'll let my group know. Sir, I'm counting on you too, you know."

As Evan hung up, he stared at the phone, wondering how Dr. Thompkins was going to be able to convince D-MACS to change course.

With all eyes on them today, any chance the panelists could hope for today would be on a wing and a prayer.

As Samantha got situated in her office, logging into her computer, she was summoned by Earl Yarborough's assistant to the CEO's office. She quickly walked over to his office and was about to open his door when Dotty stopped her.

"Mr. Yarbough is on a call but will be right with you. You can have a seat while you wait, Ms. McAllister. Can I get you anything?"

Samantha declined the offer and perched on the edge of the upholstered chair nearest Earl's office door. She caught herself chewing on one of her fingernails and forced her hands to rest on her lap. She reviewed everything in her mind as she awaited Earl.

"This weekend was a disaster. But I'm not going to let on to Earl about that. He just needs to be reassured that systems are normal and we are full speed ahead on launching this nationwide. I'm sure he just wants to confirm that. Nothing to worry about," she thought. After a couple of minutes, his door swung open.

"Ms. McAllister. Thanks for meeting with me on such short notice. Come in, come in," Earl said, smiling, as he ushered Samantha in. Once the door closed, he stopped the niceties.

"Sit. Now!"

Samantha's work was going to be cut out for her to reassure Earl that everything was fine.

"Now, I just got off the phone with a few different sources. Sounds like this weekend was a disaster. You want to tell me what the hell is going on? Or should I just take a few wild guesses?" Earl's lips thinned as he gave her a pointed look.

"I am aware of a slight hiccup that occurred but I have already addressed it. I happen to know ..."

"Listen here, Ms. McAllister. We have a lot riding on this roll out. You convinced me this initiative was going to be easy to implement and that you had everything in check. Doesn't sound like you 'happen to know' much of anything, now does it? To be perfectly frank, I'm about ready to pull the plug on this whole thing. I can just as easily be convinced to drop this and move on to other cost-saving measures. A little RIF is long overdue and would offer up a quick solution. You know, now that I think of it, I think we scrap this whole—"

"NO!" Samantha slammed her hand on Earl's desk, startling him and to some degree herself as well. She hadn't meant to let her feelings overcome her, but hearing the CEO indicate he was ready to dismiss her project was more than she could bear. She attempted to regain composure and regain his trust.

"Excuse me?"

"Sorry, sir, I mean, with all due respect. Please don't pull the plug on this yet. I would like to have one last shot at this before you decide to change course. If you'll bear with me one last time, I just know it will work. I'm willing to put my entire career on the line for this one, sir. To be perfectly honest, I did not anticipate the level of interference a few bad apples would generate. I'm going to be completely hands on with this beta test site today, and I will personally be working with one of our medical directors who will be providing the education to each of our divisions. If you'll give me twenty-four hours, I will give you the assurance you require. Please, allow me this chance? The numbers will be there. I promise."

As Samantha left the CEO's office and headed back to her office, she was seething. Earl had agreed to a twenty-four-hour reprieve, which did not leave a lot of time for her to act. Before making a call to Dr. Thompkins, she wanted to see how the panelists were scoring today. She had screamed at Theodore Butler on the drive in this morning, so she felt confident he would ensure no rogue agent activity today. But she wanted to double-check and logged on to D-MACS. Jumpy and tense, she waited for the logo to appear. Convincing herself that today, of all days, required her to be calm and focused, she decided to open up a bottle of sauvignon blanc to take the edge off. She felt warranted in this, knowing she would be cautious and just nurse the glass throughout the day.

Once logged on, she pulled up her administrative screen and awaited a chart review to transpire. As she waited, she took another sip of her wine and called Dr. Thompkins. She was already feeling more relaxed and in control thanks to the soothing effects of one of Napa's finest vintages. As the phone rang, she wondered why she had not thought of day drinking sooner. She giggled as she took another sip. After several rings, she hung up the phone.

"Oh well, I bet the old timer isn't even in the office yet. I'll call him later and set him straight." Feeling more mellow, she allowed Friday's events to fade away.

She took another sip while staring at the computer monitor. Then she got up from her office chair, glass in hand, and paced while considering her options to ensure success and to properly handle Dr. Thompkins. This would take some careful consideration.

And another sip or two of wine.

"No! I will not—so stop asking me. Neither will you, right Joanna? Tina and Charlene?"

"That's right, Keisha. I'm tired of having blood on my hands."

"I stand for what is right and I am not going to give up this fight!"

"You tell him, girl!"

Evan was not getting the unquestioned acquiescence he had hoped for. Dr. Thompkins had been very clear that they needed to stay off the radar today, and Evan was hoping to convince his group of disruptors to go along with things until the dust settled. Unfortunately, he had created a team of agitators who now felt emboldened to fight the good fight. He tried to pass around the box of donuts but got no takers.

"Listen. I hear you all loud and clear." Standing nearest the doorway to the breakroom, he leaned his head out to see if anyone was in hearing distance, especially Theo who seemed to be omnipresent today for some reason. "But we need to go through the motions today so Dr. Thompkins can take the necessary steps to get rid of this once and for all. In the meantime, he asked if we could just go with it for today. Please?"

Keisha, Joanna, Tina, and Charlene silently walked past him to exit the breakroom, Tina grabbing a sprinkled chocolate donut on her way out. Evan felt dejected and concerned. Peg tried to lift his spirits.

"Hey, that was a good try. But you did such a good job of getting them to do what is best for patients, it's going to be hard to convince them to give up their scruples now. I mean, what happens if they score without Status Quotient today? Would it complicate things?" Peg grabbed a strawberry frosted with sprinkles and took a bite.

"I ... I just don't know. I mean, look at it this way. Not all of the patients get snookered by this, right? I mean, many of them still do OK because this variable goes in their favor, right? So, let's just hope the reviews today just happen to get scored favorably, with it not being a factor anyway. I guess that's all we can hope for. And that Dr. Thompkins is able to discover a solution."

Peg smiled at Evan and squeezed his hand. "I'm sure it will work out just fine. Besides, whatever Dr. Thompkins is working on, I'm sure it will be unprecedented. I mean, the guy's a genius, yeah?"

Evan smiled back, doing his best job of trying to convince her of his confidence in the medical director. "Yeah, I'm sure whatever he has up his sleeve, it's going to be gang busters! Let's get back."

They left the breakroom and headed to their respective cubicle stations. Evan logged on just as a patient review was about to be tasked to the panelists. Evan let out a long sigh.

"C'mon, c'mon, c'mon. Let this one be an easy layup."

It wasn't.

ALL IN A DAY'S WORK

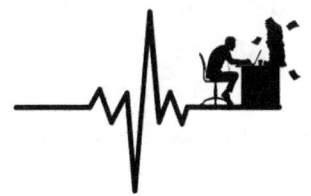

CHAPTER TWENTY

Having lived under the interstate overpass for the past several months, Rufus Jenkins was one of several homeless people who had set up camp in the inner city. He had tried shelters for years but always got kicked out for fighting or for drug use. So many rules! And Rufus thought of himself as someone who wasn't going to be told what to do. Whether or not it hurt him in the long run, he felt the freedom to do things his way at his pace was his right. Unfortunately for Rufus, things never seemed to turn out for him when doing things his way at his pace.

Unable to hold a job, he found a certain kinship in the homeless community, a group of like-minded fellow travelers going through life one day at a time. Granted, even these communities had unwritten, unsaid rules for living. For example, when Rufus happened upon several pup tents in a dumpster behind a sporting store, he didn't hoard them. Instead, he shared them with others in his group under the overpass. And take Sammy. He always seemed to come up with a surplus of canned food. So he would share and share alike. Same with Rosemarie, Bobby, Toots, and Riff Raff. Each had a talent for acquiring needed items and, like any good collective, did not mind ensuring everyone in the group was well cared for.

Unfortunately, this generosity and affinity for sharing included drug paraphernalia. The well intentions of others was often the downfall for many in the community. And Rufus, who was not known for his run of good luck, found himself on the wrong end of a needle covered with staphylococcus aureus about six weeks ago. This ended up causing a case of acute bacterial endocarditis, also known as "vegetation," on one of his heart valves. At first, he thought his fever and exhaustion were a result of the questionable found can of sardines that Riff Raff had shared with him. They had a slightly funky smell to them but, hey, they were sardines. Of course they didn't smell like roses! But since no one else in the group showed signs of food poisoning, he ruled that out. Once he saw the red rash on his hands and fingers, he worried about what was going on. The fevers at night and eventual swelling in his feet and ankles, made him finally accept help. Rosemarie, the default caretaker of the group, used a payphone to call for an ambulance.

"Come on, man, I ain't taking your money. Homeless dude? I just wouldn't feel right taking that bet. No. Uh-uh. Let's just load him up and be on our way this time, OK?" Terrell wondered if his partner had a serious gambling problem. Besides, it was getting almost impossible to know what D-MACS was going to do and where they were going to have them take the patients. It was as if they were simply flipping a coin at this point.

"You're just afraid I'm going to recoup some of my money, Shaver." Carlos's voice was goading.

"Not this time. Just double glove and come on. Grab the tackle box."

Terrell had learned long ago that responding to calls in the homeless community always put them at risk of injury, bodily harm, and infectious diseases due to the hygiene challenges faced by this population. He made it a practice to wear two pairs of latex gloves when treating a patient here, offering a minimal increase in protection from accidental needle sticks or unidentifiable body fluids.

They worked in perfect tandem, like Olympic level synchronized swimmers, Terrell thought. *Go for the gold.* They made quick work of assessing the patient and had him loaded on the stretcher and heading toward the back of the ambulance in record time. As Carlos pushed, Terrell made the call to dispatch.

"Dispatch, this is Shaver. We got a fifty-seven-year-old homeless gentleman. Temp 103.6. Heart rate 126. Blood pressure low, 80s over 40s. He's got a rash on his hands, palms, and fingers. Swollen feet and ankle bilaterally. History of IV drug use. No other health history that we can discern. Over."

"Shaver, this is Central Dispatch, copy that. Got a name? Over."

"Sir? What's your name? Sir? Yes, you. What's your name?" The man mumbled his name.

"OK. Thanks, man." He returned to his radio. "Dispatch,

we have a Rufus Jenkins here. Where we heading? Over."

"Shaver, we are uploading the info now. Go ahead and load up the patient. I'll get back to you about your destination before you even get behind the wheel. Over."

Terrell and Carlos finished loading Rufus into the back of the ambulance when Terrell got notification from Central.

"Shaver, this is Central Dispatch. You're not going to believe this. Head to Regional General with lights and siren. Over."

Terrell turned to Carlos and shrugged.

Didn't see that coming.

Dr. Thompkins and Dr. Corneal continued to debate potential solutions, never coming any closer to an agreeable decision. Either the answer was not decisive enough to make what they deemed as necessary changes or was too strong and would have disastrous downstream effects. They had been deliberating all weekend and were still no closer to coming up with a way to turn things around.

It didn't help matters that they were both scared of what next steps Samantha McAllister would do if provoked. She had already scared Simon into hiding.

"Just to make things worse, I guess now is as good a time as any to let you know I told Evan this morning that I would let him know of the plan today."

"Why would you tell him that? We've hit a brick wall. And you're supposed to do live-video education nationwide to each district, what, in three days? There's no way. No way at all."

"Well, what would happen if we didn't find an agreed upon remedy? Just for argument's sake. What if this did go nationwide? Then what?"

Simon stared at his colleague. "Seriously? You're asking me? You know what would happen, better than I do, Harold. We are talking about a medical catastrophe of biblical proportions. And I'm not being hyperbolic, either, mind you. This would be the denial of necessary healthcare on a level that we have never seen in our lifetime. I can't sit by idly and watch the world I've come to know and care for just crumble around me. I won't. I just won't, Harold." Simon's eyes teared up.

"OK, OK. We agree. This cannot happen. Our entire careers will be upended, and everything we've worked for would go *pfft*, just like that. No, no. We'll think of something. But it's got to be decisive, and it's got to move us forward and not backward."

Just then, the phone rang. Recognizing the number, Dr. Thompkins told Simon, "It's Samantha again. She's tenacious if nothing else."

"You're going to have to talk to her at some point, Harold. Just get it over with. Maybe she'll say something that helps us decide here."

Dr. Thompkins answered the phone on the fifth ring. "Well hello, Ms. McAllister, I was just going to call you back. I'm so sorry I missed your other calls earlier, I had some conflicting meetings that were more pressing. But now I'm here. How can I help you?"

She berated him for two solid minutes, with him holding the receiver at arm's length from his ear for much of the time. Finally, when she began winding down, he returned the phone to his ear. "I truly am sorry about that. I must have gotten the dates wrong. They seemingly do them all the time, so I didn't look closely. That was an innocent mistake on my part, Ms. McAllister. Innocent, indeed. However, I can assure you, my modifications to the presentation I am doing in a few days are almost complete. I am certainly looking forward to getting this project off the ground, nationwide." Dr. Thompkins rolled his eyes at Simon.

Simon returned the gesture by pretending to stick his finger down his throat and make himself throw up.

"A new score just came in, you say? Well, I'm sure it is ... Ms. McAllister. Please stop yelling. I can't understand ... Ms. McAllister. What is it you are saying?"

Dr. Thompkins stared at the receiver then hung the phone up.

"What was that all about?"

"Well, she hung up on me. She started shouting about a new score as posted by the panelists that was going to result in an IV-drug-using homeless person getting top tier treatment. At least that's what it sounded like she was saying. Surely she was mistaken though. I mean, I just spoke with Evan this morning. He wouldn't have sent up any alarm bells today of all days, would he?"

Dr. Thompkins logged into D-MACS and pulled up the just-tabbed patient chart review. He reviewed the notes and chart for a moment, then slumped back in his chair.

"Simon, our day of reckoning has come. She is going to go DEFCON one on this, I tell you. If we don't find the solution, like right this instant, then I think we'll have no choice but to get drastic."

Simon and Dr. Thompkins stared at each other, shaking their heads. Dr. Thompkins hoped and prayed for a miracle solution.

But would it be in time?

Theo liked Mondays. He knew he was in the minority, but he always felt that the start of a new work week arrived with hope and opportunity. With little to interest him during his off time, he thought of his team of panelists as family and looked forward to seeing them each week. Well, to be fair, he looked forward to seeing *most* of them each week. He knew Murray was back today after his suspension and wasn't sure what mood he would be in on return. Noticing that Evan had brought in donuts for the team, however, gave Theo hope that, quite possibly, today was going to be a good day.

Then the phone rang and he saw the caller ID.

Bracing himself for impact, he picked up the receiver. "Good morning, Ms. McAllister. Happy Monday!" Theo felt Monday-morning patter should be enjoyed by everyone.

"THIS ENDS NOW!"

"Um, I'm not exactly sure what you are referring to, Ms. McAllister. What is 'ending'?"

"Well, let's start with your incompetence as a shift supervisor. How else would you explain the scoring that was just submitted?"

"I, um, actually have not had a chance to review the chart you are referring to ... let me ... um ... log in and ..."

"You can review all you want. But I am coming down there, mister, and I am going to take this bull by the horns and end the rebelliousness and cavalier attitude of your panelists NOW! Do you hear me? I have put up with your ineptitude for the last time! I will be there in ten minutes. Be ready."

Click.

Theo felt the blood drain from his face as he hung up the phone.

"What did they do? What did they do?" Theo repeated, pulling up the most recently tabbed chart, one belonging to a Rufus Jenkins. A number of panelists had mis-scored the review. He sank in his chair, not knowing what to do. Theo's clumsy attempts to manage the panelists had obviously fallen on deaf ears, and he understood better the reason for Samantha's ire. Feeling he had to show that he had done something, anything, and hopefully offset Ms. McAllister's wrath, he decided to call a mandatory meeting for all the panelists. Maybe if she arrived on the floor and saw him raking them over the coals, she might take some sympathy on him.

It was a small chance, but, hey … Mondays were full of hope and optimism, right?

Evan couldn't help rubbernecking a few times. Murray was doubled over in his office chair, clutching his abdomen. Despite the space between them, Evan could hear the loud rumblings coming from Murray's midsection. In fact, the gurgling witch's cauldron that was Murray's stomach sounded like it was going to explode at any minute.

"Psst. Hey, Putz. I don't know what was in that bear claw, but I'm dying here. Cover for me, will ya?"

Murray then made a beeline to the men's room, still hunched over, obviously trying to hold on to the gastric contents that were preparing to see the light of day once again.

Evan thought to himself, "Maybe, Murr, maybe it was the rancid milk still in your coffee cup this morning. Jeez." As Murray hustled to the restroom, Theo made his way around the corner, his face angry and determined.

"Mandatory meeting in the conference room. Now! C'mon, that means everyone!" He spun and stomped off in the direction of the conference room.

Everyone slowly got up from their workstations, looking clueless and probably trying to figure out the cause of Theo's rare outburst.

Evan, on the other hand, was fairly certain he knew what was going on. He caught Peg's eye and she nodded toward Keisha, Joanna, Tina, and Charlene as they saddled up to them on the way to the called meeting.

"I told you all that Dr. Thompkins asked us to 'stay off the radar' today!" Evan kept his voice down as they approached the conference room. "What did you do? Did you screw up the last review?"

Keisha, Joanna, Tina, and Charlene eyed each other, shrugged in unison, then quietly filed into the room.

Theo, standing in front of a bunch of chairs, paused after everyone had filed in and taken seats. "Where is Murray? Anyone know where Murray is?"

Evan raised his hand. "Um, I think you are going to want

to start without him. He might be indisposed for a while, if you know what I mean."

Several people snickered.

"OK, OK. Enough of that. Evan, catch him up with what he missed."

As Theo proceeded to lecture them on the importance of their work and the white-hot laser-focus that was on them as a beta testing site for Status Quotient, Evan had a hard time not mentally checking out. He sensed that this sermon given by Reverend Theodore Butler was going to be a long one, starting at Genesis and going right through Revelation. Everyone else appeared just as bleary-eyed as he felt.

"We have been chosen to test this new calculation, and we will not let the company down!"

"Each of you must take this seriously!"

"I am asking, no, I am *commanding* each of you to realize the gravity of your role here."

Peg elbowed Evan just as he did a head bob.

He whispered to her, "What do you expect of me? Two donuts, an overcrowded meeting room, and Theo's monotone droning? Night, night."

"Now," Theo went on, "we are going to review the first case tabbed by each of you this morning, line by line, word by word, to ensure you are all on the same page."

This was crazy. He couldn't keep them captive here all day in the conference room, could he? Evan almost wished he were Murray and thus avoiding this purgatory.

Almost.

"**Eureka!**" Dr. Thompkins shouted and grabbed his keys.

Simon jumped up. "You got a plan? Tell me!"

"I can't believe I didn't think of this sooner. I'm going to plead our case to Earl Yarborough. As CEO, he needs to hear from the voice of reason how this new initiative is going to result in blood on his hands. Lord knows he's obviously not going to get that from Samantha. I mean, I've still got some pull around here. Hell, I'm the medical director for crying out loud. If he won't listen to me, then heaven help us all. Want to come? Two are better than one, right?"

"I better not. I've never met the guy and to be perfectly honest with you, I'd rather not run into Samantha, you know?"

Dr. Thompkins tapped his finger to his temple. "Smart man. I didn't think about that. Yes, that would be quite the explosion on the Fourth of July. How about you log on and keep tabs on any more chart reviews that pop up. That way we can be proactive with any aberrant scoring before Samantha does. Wish me luck!"

Simon stood up and shook Dr. Thompkins's hand. "I'm proud to be here, sharing this moment with you, Harold. This is monumental. John Q. Public has no idea of the atom bomb that will be unleashed if we don't stop this. If YOU don't stop this. We have a literal chance to change history, here. I mean, when we were practicing at the bedside, we would save, what, one life at a time? This is our opportunity to save the lives of tens of thousands. Be strong. Be courageous. And be convincing!"

Dr. Thompkins smiled back. "Thanks, Simon. I'm proud of you too, old friend. You're right. We have been given this opportunity to stop a train from careening off the track, trying to take the lives of thousands of innocents along with it. I'll call you as soon as I'm finished."

He left his office and made his way down to the street. A light rain fell, so he turned up the collar on his coat and hurried as best he could to his parked car. Once inside, he started it up and turned on the windshield wipers and defrost to clear his view. This gave him a moment to offer up a silent prayer, one that put his entire faith on the line to be heard. Easing his way into traffic, he felt a sudden pressure to get to the CEO's office as soon as possible. Knowing the voraciousness of Samantha McAllister's desire to be successful, he sensed that if he didn't get his voice heard soon, all hope would be lost.

Dr. Thompkins weaved in and out of traffic, driving faster than he normally would in these conditions, hurried along by his sense of justice. His Lexus sedan cut off other drivers, and he ran more than one red light as he sped through the city on his way to his destiny. As he drove across the intersection of 15th Street and Lexington, all four tires actually left the road as he flew over the crosswalks.

The closer he came to his destination, the faster he drove. Adrenaline coursing through his veins, his breathing was short and labored. His accelerated heart rate matched his revved up 3.4-liter V6 engine. He was on a mission and nothing was going to get in his way.

That was his plan, anyway.

After slamming the phone down on Theodore Butler, Samantha finished off her most-recently poured glass of wine. Then she grabbed her coat, purse, and keys. Once her lipstick was reapplied in the mirror, she turned off her computer and raced toward the elevator. Looking back on her work history, she strained to recall working with a more amateurish group. From her years interning in Congress, she was familiar with a certain level of inefficiency and foot dragging, but that seemed to be more intentional in order to delay the passing of bills or mobilization of differing factions. This, on the other hand? This was just a complete bungling of one absurdity after another.

As she rode the elevator down to the parking deck, she considered her options with how to best handle Theo. His impotent management style had probably been overlooked for years with the way D-MACS had been led in the past. Now, with the firestorm of Samantha McAllister at the helm, his ineffectual leadership must go. And the same went for the aging medical director, Dr. Thompkins. His antiquated style and outdated ideas needed to be mothballed and perhaps set up in the Smithsonian for historical preservation. His ways may have worked in the past, but not in these days of rapid cycle change, baby.

"Lead, follow, or get out the way you old coot!" Samantha said out loud as she walked through the parking deck, slightly louder than she had intended. She doublechecked to make sure no one had noticed her outburst. She unlocked her car and quickly started up her Porsche 911, revving the twin-turbocharged 3.7-liter engine to ensure anyone within earshot knew she was ready to kick ass. She squealed out of her parking space and wound around the parking deck towards the exit. As she exploded onto the city streets, she switched on her windshield wipers to combat the moderate rain blanketing the city.

Thinking about how close Theo had come to derailing her plans for implementation caused Samantha such indigestion that she coughed up a small amount of bile. She used a tissue to remove the bitter yellow green expectorant from her mouth. Blaming the shift supervisor as well as the medical director's incompetence for this physical manifestation, Samantha grew more enraged. She weaved in and out of traffic, hurried faster by her sense of vengeance. Her Porsche 911 darted between drivers, prompting the honking of horns and multiple one-finger salutes.

The closer Samantha came to the panelists' office building, the faster she drove. Several times she had to use the back of her hand to wipe off the windshield, which kept fogging up from her rapid breathing. Her pounding heart rate was slow and methodical compared to the speeding of her sports car through the city streets. She was bound and determined to show Theodore Butler who was boss and nothing was going to get in her way.

That was her plan, anyway.

Murray finally felt well enough to brave the real world and meandered back to his cubicle. It had been a while since he was on the business end of food poisoning and vowed to never eat a baked offering from Evan ever again. "He probably got it from the trash, the jerk." Back at his desk, he caught onto the silence and wondered where everyone was. He stuck his head out of his cubicle to see and noticed the conference room door was open. Inside, Theo was pointing at a computer, all red-faced and speaking furiously. Office meeting.

"I'll pass." Murray said to himself. "Besides, I gotta be close to homebase if that nasty bear claw rears its ugly head again." After lowering himself to his office chair, he logged onto his workstation and stared at the D-MACS logo on the home screen. "It's just as well. I've been lectured by Theo more than my share the past few days." He slowly rubbed his stomach as he tried to will himself toward feeling better. It didn't help, so he added in some low sympathy moans. "Uhhh. Uhhh. Uhhh." They didn't help but they didn't hurt either. As he was the only panelist on the floor at the time, no one seemed to mind his attempts at improved health.

"Uhhh. Uhhh."

Other drivers did their best to avoid the dangerous maneuvering of the fast-moving car on the rain slicked asphalt. The velocity reached speeds that would make a professional racecar driver say, "Slow down!" But there were times in one's life where caution was thrown to the wind and a person's id overpowered their more cautious superego. This could be a noble exercise, especially when seen through the lens of history where the outcome resulted in a satisfactory ending. In reality, though, reckless behavior in the face of fixed obstacles such as increasingly rainy conditions, less skilled drivers, distracted pedestrians, or, as in this case, a large garbage truck that had come to a complete stop, could oftentimes put a quick end to the best of intentions. The speeding car, many times lighter than the twenty-ton behemoth making its scheduled trash pickups, had little chance of coming out of the collision unscathed. The only bright spot was that the expensive car was designed with safety in mind, regardless of the irresponsible navigation of the driver. The airbags deployed in less than 1/20th of a second, giving first responders a chance to provide first aid until the ambulance could arrive. The rain let up a bit, allowing onlookers the chance to see that the driver was still breathing and able to respond to urgent pleas to "Hold on" and "Help is coming." But help would need to arrive awfully quick.

When D-MACS developed the determination of healthcare by chart reviews done by panelists years ago, the tabulation calculated an aggregate score, throwing out, essentially, the highest or lowest score, and coming up with an average that was done by several members of the team. This was a safety net which was carefully added. Over the years, many other safety steps were created in order to provide proper oversight and uniformity amongst the panelists.

When D-MACS introduced Status Quotient in the beta testing site, however, several important safety layers were removed, one of which was the minimum-number body-count for panelists. And this morning, Murray was flying solo.

It wasn't Murray's job to worry about being the sole reviewer of the motor vehicle accident listed on his computer. He was sure D-MACS had some protocol in place to allow for it. For Murray, he was going through the motions as much as he could with a stomach that felt like it was attempting to turn inside out. If the developer of Status Quotient had better foresight, then this safety net most certainly would not have been removed. But as the kids said, "It is what it is."

Arriving on the scene, Terrell and Carlos were faced with pure carnage. Having responded to hundreds of motor vehicle accidents, they had seen some doozies in their time. This one ranked up there as being one of the dooziest. After grabbing their gear, they made their way to the crumpled metal frame and made a path through the well-wishers and good Samaritans so as to assess the situation. They made quick work of providing trauma care as best as they could in the light rain and metal debris field. Carlos got the IV going and initiated a couple liter bags of fluid to maintain a blood pressure in light of the obvious loss of blood at the scene. Eventually, they were able to load onto the stretcher while Terrell called it in.

"Dispatch, this is Shaver. We got a pretty gnarly MVA here. I can't get a temp read, but heart rate is 130s, blood pressure is low 90s over 50s. Large amount of bleeding at the site and, based on presentation, I'm putting money on at least a ruptured spleen, possibly a lacerated liver due to a right abdominal puncture from part of the car frame. We're on our second liter of LR and want to know where to head. Oh, and one more thing I guess I should mention. Over."

"Copy that. What else, Shaver? Over."

Terrell paused for a moment.

"This one smells like a brewery. Over."

"Copy that, Shaver. Got a name? Over."

"Got her wallet right here—hang on a sec. OK, here's the license. Dispatch, we have a Samantha McAllister here. Where are we heading? Over."

"Uploading the info now. Load up and I'll let you know where you're going in a jiffy. Over."

Terrell and Carlos rolled the stretcher over to their truck and got Samantha placed in the ambulance.

The call came back quick over the radio. "Shaver, this is Central Dispatch. I tell you, I don't know what is what anymore. Looks like you are not only heading to Shady Grove Community Hospital on the north side of town, but you've been instructed to not use lights or siren and to go ahead and stop the IV fluids. Over."

"Shady Grove. Shady Grove. Man, we haven't been up there in months. That's the small hospital with the barbeque restaurant nearby, ain't it, Dispatch? Over."

"That's the one. The Puckered Pig. Their BBQ sauce will knock your socks off. Enjoy! Over."

Terrell and Carlos slowly made their way through the police cars and tow truck that was already trying to load up the crumpled ball of a Porche 911. Only lunchtime, and they'd already had a long day.

Carlos begrudgingly handed Terrell a twenty-dollar bill.

"Keep it, Carlos. How 'bout this? Lunch is on you. Sound good?"

"Sounds good, my man. How long 'til we get there? I'm starving!"

"GPS says about an hour, an hour and a half, depending on traffic and this rain. Let's put on some tunes and enjoy the ride, buddy."

Singing along as Foghat's "Slow Ride" filled the speakers in the ambulance, Terrell and Carlos made their way to the north side of town.

After parking his car, Dr. Thompkins hurried up to the CEO's office. It had been a few years since he had last made his way to this office building. Noticing the leather furniture and upscale light fixtures, he assumed those at this level of D-MACS were not hurting for money. Upon exiting the elevator, he walked to Earl's office and made his way to the assistant's desk.

The woman smiled. "Excuse me, sir, may I help you?" Her name plate read "Dotty."

"Oh, hi there. Um, yes, I am Dr. Thompkins, medical director at D-MACS. I need to speak with Mr. Yarborough urgently. This is a matter of life and death." Dr. Thompkins had practiced this repeatedly on the drive over and thought it sounded the most concise yet conveyed a keen sense of urgency.

"I'm sure it is very important that you speak with Mr. Yarborough, but you will need to have an appointment."

"Now see here. I simply must speak with him, right this minute. Did you not hear me about this being a matter of life and death?"

"Oh, I heard you, Doctor. Unfortunately, Mr. Yarborough is not in at the moment. Could I set up a day and time for you to meet with him?" She covered a yawn with her hand.

"I'll just go to him then. Tell me. Where is Earl Yarborough? I must see him today."

"Sir, you seem like a nice enough guy. I'll just schedule you a day and time. How about"—she looked at her computer screen— "a week from next Tuesday? He's got a 10:15 and a 3:45 available."

"Am I speaking gibberish? No, I *don't* want an appointment. I am demanding you tell me where he is. I will go to him and plead my case." Dr. Thompkins did his best to stand upright and appear immovable.

Letting out a sigh, Dotty leaned in and motioned for Dr. Thompkins to come closer.

"Listen, you didn't hear it from me, OK? But there is a boat show in town, and Mr. Yarborough likes to go each year to figure out which one he wants to upgrade to. If you want to see him so badly, I'd suggest you make your way over there."

Dr. Thompkins was dumbfounded. He felt both defeated and deflated. With a feeble smile at Dotty, he thanked her. Then, slowly, he walked away toward the bank of elevators. With the weight of the world on his shoulders, he was positive that, if allowed, he could just collapse into a crumpled heap. Once in his car, he thought about calling Simon to break the bad news but decided it would be better to let him know in person that he was unable to meet with the CEO of D-MACS.

Taking the long way back to his office, he used his time in the car to debate whether he should resign his position as medical director immediately and just go back into private practice or retire completely and put the woes of healthcare behind him. After parking the car, he headed into his office. Upon exiting the elevator at his floor, he could hear shouts coming from inside his office. He quickly unlocked the door, expecting to find Simon in a heated brawl with an intruder. Instead, he found Simon on the phone.

Smiling.

THE ONLY CONSTANT
IN LIFE IS CHANGE

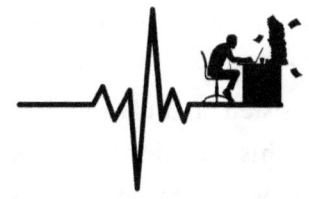

CHAPTER TWENTY-ONE

"For he's a jolly good fell-OOOOOOO
That nobody can deny!"
Harry held up his glass of tonic water with lime to give a toast.

"Everyone, everyone—I'd like to say a few words about my nephew if you will all indulge me. Here is to one of the hardest working, most dedicated guys I've ever had the pleasure of knowing. I am confident it is due to his tireless commitment to doing the 'right thing' that has resulted in his promotion to shift supervisor! I am also proud to say that he has inherited all of my best attributes: he's caring, smart as a whip, and as handsome as the day is long! Evan—here is to you, my fine nephew! May you have all the happiness and luck that life can hold!"

"Cheers!"

"Here's to Evan!"

"Hooray!"

Sitting next to Peg, Evan beamed and took a sip of his

drink. Several well-wishers patted him on the back, and he was somewhat surprised by the turnout for his promotion celebration. Most of his fellow panelists had come to celebrate, including Peg, Keisha, Joanna, Tina, Charlene ... and even Murray. Dr. Thompkins and Dr. Simon Corneal were here as well, having a lively debate in a side booth. Harry was the one who had insisted on throwing the impromptu party to make the most of his achievement. When Peg had let him know of the promotion, Harry took the news and ran with it.

"You're not mad at me are you? I just knew Harry would be thrilled to hear of you becoming the new shift supervisor. And so am I!" Peg leaned on her barstool and gave Evan an excited hug.

"Nah, I'm OK with it. I mean, I've never liked being the center of attention, but when you got the goods ..." Evan drifted off as he pretended to kiss his biceps. "... I guess it goes with the territory, you know?"

They laughed at the same time and hugged again.

He drew back and nodded towards the small crowd. "Hey, I guess I better make some rounds. You good? Do you need another drink?"

"No, I'm good." She grinned at him. "I'll be right here making sure Harry doesn't get into any trouble."

Harry, hearing his name, lit up and came over to the barstools where Peg and Evan were sitting.

"I'm proud of you, Squirt. I knew you had it in you! Here, let me top off that drink of yours."

Evan placed his palm over his glass. "No, Harry. I'm good. I don't want to get too crazy as the new shift supervisor, you know? But thanks, seriously. Thanks for everything."

Harry grinned at him. "Smart, good looking and the consummate professional to boot. A triple threat!"

Evan went around, thanking his friends and co-workers for joining in on the festivities. Keisha, Joanna, Tina, and Charlene were huddled together, chatting up a storm. When Evan approached, they shouted and welcomed him over.

"No hard feelings, right? Mr. Shift Supervisor?"

"We just had to follow our instincts and do the right thing in fighting the power, you know what I'm saying?"

"You know, if we *hadn't* scored the homeless guy so low last week, none of this would have happened, right?"

"I mean, if you were shift supervisor, we wouldn't have done anything, you know that, right Evan?"

"Wait, wait, wait. You mean it was YOU guys who made Theo so mad we had to listen to him in that sweat tank of a conference room for hours? I knew it! Why didn't you admit to it earlier?"

"We thought you'd be mad at us, Evan. But we're all good now, right? It all worked out the way it was supposed to, anyway."

"Isn't that right, Mr. Shift Supervisor?"

Together, the four of them offered up their hands as if in prayer.

"Pleeeease?"

Evan smiled at them. "Of course I'm not mad. I just wish I was as strong in my convictions as you all are. You're amazing panelists, and I'm glad you are all on my team. This is going to be great!"

They each said "Cheers" to Evan then resumed their huddle to chat as he made his way around the rest of the room. As he approached the solitary figure, he felt almost sorry for him. Almost.

"Thanks for coming, Murr. I didn't think you would."

"Don't be getting a big head or anything, Putz. I just came in for a drink. I didn't know of any 'celebration' or anything." Murray glared at Evan. Then winked. "I'm just kidding. Man! You should see your face. Of course ol' Murr is going to be here. I'm the life of the party, after all!"

Evan let out a sigh as he realized, for the first time, that being the shift supervisor for the panelists meant *all* the panelists. Including Murray. *Sigh.* "Of course you are, Murr! I hope we can let all bygones be bygones. Can you do that?" He held out his hand.

Murray grabbed his chin in thought, then smiled and shook Evan's hand. "Of course! Ol' Murr doesn't hold grudges, you know that." Then, pulling Evan in closer, he became stern and glared at Evan. "Just don't bring in any of those rancid bear claws again, got it, boss?" He let out a classic Murray laugh.

After agreeing to Murray's demands, he went to see Dr. Thompkins, the one who had made it all happen.

It turned out Dr. Thompkins had made several recommendations (some might have said they were requirements for his agreement to stay on as medical director) to Earl Yarborough. They were immediately accepted and implemented. One was the swift removal of Theodore Butler. The entire floor (sans Murray) had signed a complaint against Theo after the mandatory three-and-a-half-hour meeting in the conference room. The grievances sent to HR included "false imprisonment," "slanderous accusations," "hints of retaliation," "overall malice intimidation," and (this was a bit of a stretch but it was listed on the complaint) "deleterious effects resulting from hyperthermia exposure." (It was hot in the conference room!)

Rather than go through the arduous process of investigating each complaint and getting statements from each panelist, Dr. Thompkins made the decision to relieve Theo of his duties, effective immediately, and promote Evan to the role of shift supervisor. Rumor had it when Theo was notified of this decision, he burst into tears and sobbed, "Thank you, thank you, thank you!" to the HR generalist who was on the phone. A joint decision had been made to move him to HR for hiring and recruitment, under the tutelage of Richard Brannigan. Theo was delighted to be moved to a change of scenery.

"I just wanted to thank you again, Dr. Thompkins, for the recommendation and your confidence in me for the promotion. I won't let you down. I promise."

Dr. Thompkins smiled up at Evan. "I know you will do a wonderful, wonderful job. You know, Simon and I haven't had a chance to thank you for your leadership with the rest of the panelists over the last few weeks. If it weren't for you and your steadfast determination to do what was right, I'm not sure how this would have all turned out. But you, young man, you stuck to your guns and made a difference. Knowing that good guys still exist out there gives old timers like me and Simon hope."

Simon had appeared at Dr. Thompkins's elbow. "Hey! Speak for yourself, calling me an 'old timer.' I'm a good three years younger than you, Harold! But, yes, I would like to echo my aging colleague in his praise of the risk you took in taking on 'the machine.' True heroes are hard to find these days, you know. But you ... you should think about getting a cape, Evan!"

Evan glowed as he basked in the accolades from his respected medical friends. "Thank you so much. I have to tell you, I don't think I could have done it alone." Evan waved at Peg and urged her to come over.

As Peg approached, Evan smiled. "Peg here is the one you should be heaping praise on. To be perfectly honest with you, if it weren't for her, I doubt I would have had the conviction to do any of the things that transpired. Peg here ... well, she's the real hero."

"Ah, yes indeed, she is something special," said Dr. Thompkins.

Dr. Thompkins and Simon both offered their hands for a shake.

Peg turned the color of a ripe tomato. "Oh, my goodness! I'm speechless. Thank you! I am truly without words. You are all so sweet!"

As Peg and Evan walked away from the physicians, the two doctors resumed their philosophical debate. Evan felt lighthearted—if anyone could solve the problems of this world, good money would be on these guys.

"I'm so embarrassed, Evan!" She covered her face. "I didn't do anything!"

Evan turned to her, took both of her hands in his and met her gaze. "You believed in me. You gave me courage. I was really struggling at one point with my work. Hell, ask Harry someday. But you came along and you made me feel like I could make a difference. And we, WE did it, Peg. WE made a difference after all!"

Peg reached up and held Evan's face in her hands, tears spilling onto her cheeks. Gazing into each other's eyes, they were silent for several seconds, before both gushing "I love you!" at the exact same time. They then kissed, consummating their declaration to each other. And, by the way, it was a good kiss. A really good kiss. Evan's heart raced.

Harry, always the perfect host, somehow saw this coming a mile away because he was standing next to them when they opened their eyes, holding two glasses of champagne.

"Peg. Evan. What a cute couple! I just can't hardly stand it! Here, please, a glass of champagne for the two of you. Toast one another and let's get this party started!"

Evan and Peg raised their champagne flutes to each other, clinking them together before taking a sip. In the background, singing started. First it was Harry leading the way; then, the whole bar joined in as Kool and the Gang's "Celebration" reverberated off the walls.

Back at work the next week, Dr. Thompkins spent a few extra minutes preparing his pipe before reading the morning paper. After ensuring that the tobacco was properly packed, he lit a match and puffed his pipe into a fine working order. He then opened up the paper and went to his favorite section. Reviewing the names listed to ensure there was no one he knew, he stopped abruptly and read the most recent obituary listing with a combination of sadness mixed with a smoldering of relief.

"Samantha McAllister was laid to rest after a tragic automobile accident. Her dedication to the betterment of others was obvious to all who had the good fortune of knowing her. She was hard-working and was a devoted change agent with D-MACS. She was known by all around her to put others first, especially those who were considered less fortunate. This philanthropic philosophy of hers was her guiding light in a world full of darkness. She could be counted on to give to those in need, saying her favorite quote, "There, but for the grace of God, go I" as she would drop a spare coin into a tin cup. In lieu of flowers, please send donations to your favorite homeless shelter. That's what Samantha would have wanted."

That's it? Nothing about trying to eradicate mankind one patient at a time? Seriously? He dropped the paper back on his desk and sent up a fresh smoke ring toward the light fixture above his head. His laughter bubbled out. At first he felt guilty for finding humor in someone's passing. But the irony of it all was just too much for him. And he laughed and laughed and laughed.

The good Lord sure did work in mysterious ways, didn't He?

Terrell and Carlos were glad to have more predictability in their work again. Gone were the surprises and the randomness of each call. Oh, there were still the calls that made them scratch their heads, with a seemingly never-ending supply of crazy out there. But at least they could now, with better confidence, know what D-MACS was going to do with each patient. They unanimously gave up on betting on which hospital Dispatch was going to send them to. They felt they had moved past that type of thing. It had always left them with a bad feeling anyways.

As they pulled up to the house where 9-1-1 had been called, the new betting began.

"No socks, no shoes. Twenty dollars. I just know it! I can feel it! Hell, I can smell it!"

"Bare feet? That means nothing but feet. If they have on flip-flops, that counts as shoes, right?"

"Man! Flip flops ain't' no shoes. Uh-uh. If you can see the toes, then it ain't a shoe."

"Of course they're shoes. You wear them so you can walk around and not step in crap. Counts as a shoe. Take it or leave it."

Carlos thought about it. He eyed the house and then saw the upholstered couch on the front porch and several cars without tires in the front yard.

"I'll take it. You are a sucker, Terrell! Just look at the couch! I mean, someone puts a couch on the porch, they're not gonna be wearing socks and shoes. That's science talkin', not me. Science!"

"OK, OK. But it's gotta be the patient, this time. Having some baby with no socks and shoes on doesn't count. The bet is on the patient, right?"

They shook hands then got out of the ambulance.

After they got their gear from the truck, they made their way to the door of the house. They were ushered almost immediately into where the patient lay prone on the floor. No shoes. One sock on.

Terrell smiled as Carlos slipped him the twenty.

It's been a long time since Terrell lost a bet. A long time.

THE END

www.ingramcontent.com/pod-product-compliance
Lightning Source LLC
Chambersburg PA
CBHW071540110726
47908CB00007B/1950